BEGINNER'S WORKOUT PROGRAMS FOR SPECIFIC GOALS

A 30 days fat Burning Challenge for Total beginners without heavy gym equipment for exercise.

Dr. Diana S. Weatherall

TABLE OF CONTENTS

INTRODUCTION

Welcome to the journey of transformation! I'm thrilled to share this practical guide for beginners, born out of my personal quest for fitness and well-being.No fluff, no complicated routines – just a clear, straightforward actionable plan based on my personal journey and success stories approach to help you kickstart your own fitness journey.

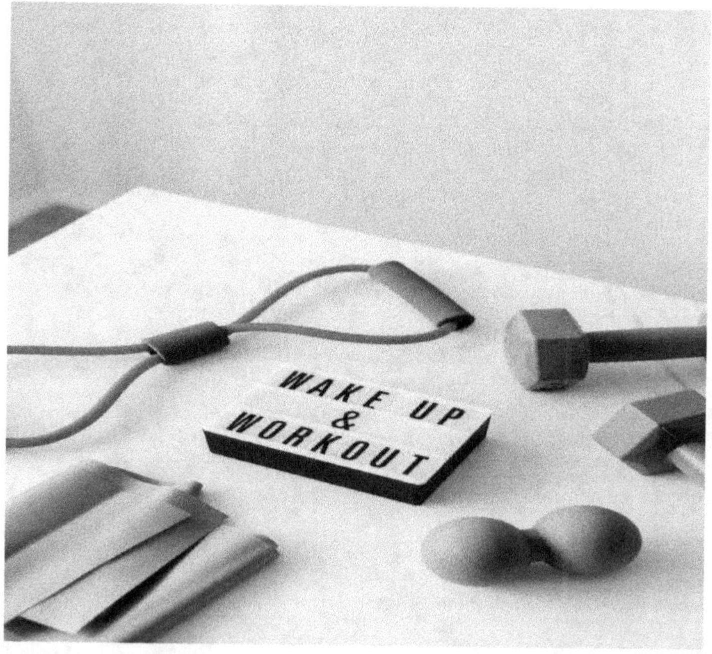

A few years back, I found myself overwhelmed with conflicting advice, intimidating gym equipment, and a longing for a healthier lifestyle. I vividly remember the day I stared at a gym schedule like it was an alien language, feeling lost amidst the sea of weights and cardio machines.

But from that confusion emerged a simple idea – a beginner-friendly workout program tailored to specific goals. As I stumbled through my own fitness journey, learning from missteps and celebrating small victories, I realized the need for a guide that demystifies the world of fitness for beginners.

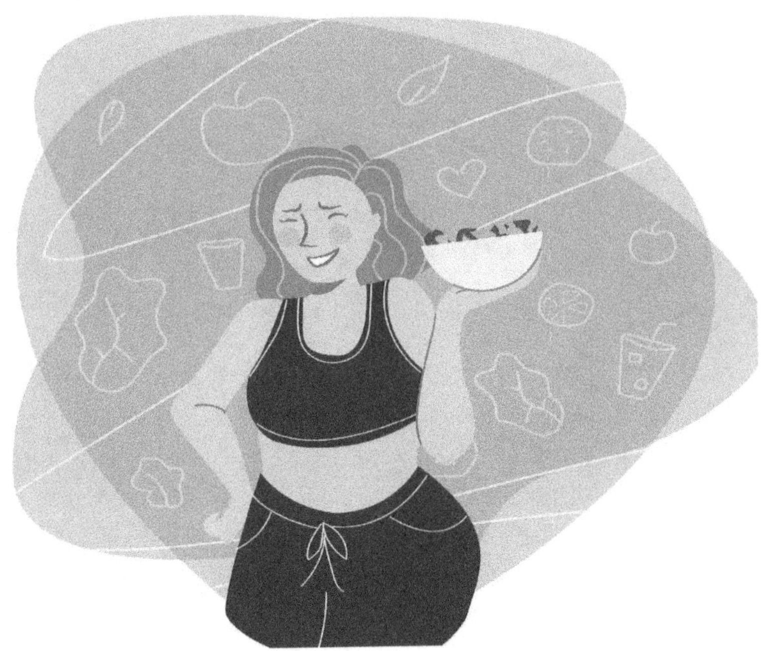

In these pages, I'll share stories of my struggles, breakthroughs, and the lessons learned along the way. You don't need to be an athlete or a fitness guru to understand and apply the principles outlined here. Whether your goal is strength, toning, or just improving overall fitness, this book is your companion.

Now, let's embark on this journey together. Flip the page, lace up those sneakers, and let's make strides toward a healthier, stronger you. Your journey begins here – let's make it extraordinary!

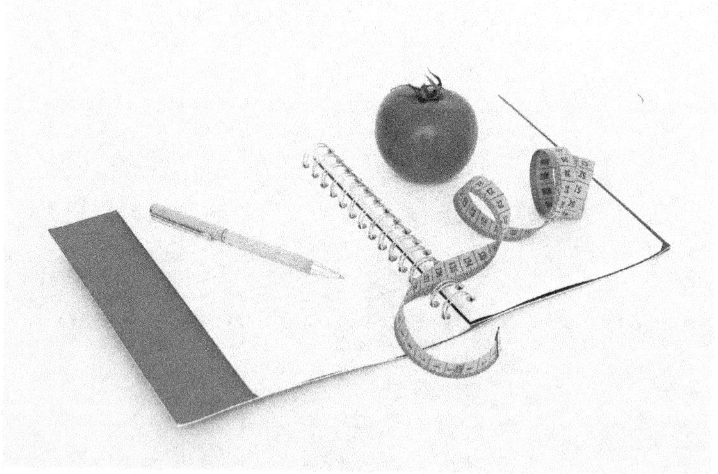

CHAPTER 1

1.1: UNDERSTANDING YOUR GOALS

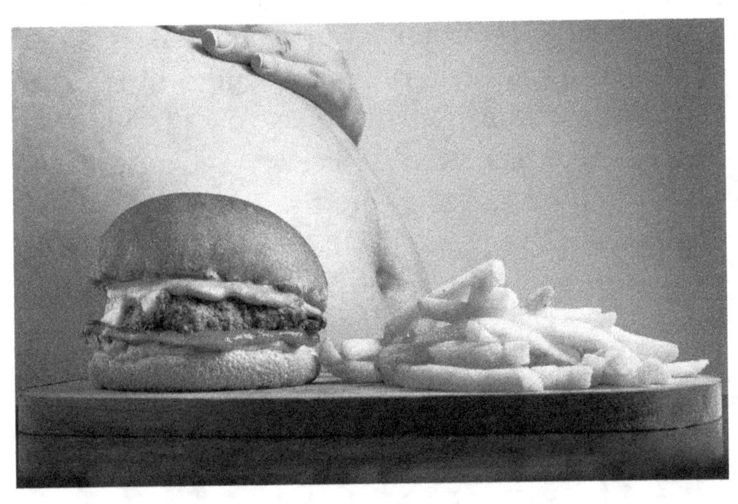

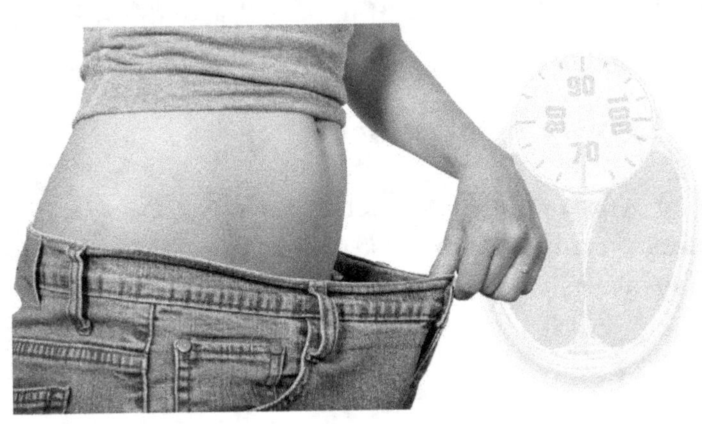

Embarking on a fitness journey is like stepping into a realm of possibilities, and my journey started with a challenge – a 30-day Fat Burning Challenge designed for total beginners, no equipment needed. Picture this: a month of workouts that required nothing more than determination and a little space in my living room. Let me take you through this transformative experience as we delve into the essence of understanding your fitness goals.

1. The Spark of a Challenge

It all began with a desire for change, a whisper of, "Can I do this?" The challenge presented itself as a roadmap – a structured plan for someone who was clueless about where to start. Thirty days of commitment sounded daunting, yet the simplicity of the challenge drew me in. No gym, no fancy equipment – just me, a timer, and a willingness to embrace change.

2. The Power of a Defined Goal

In the world of fitness, setting a clear goal is like turning on a light in a dark room. The goal for these 30 days was straightforward – burn fat.

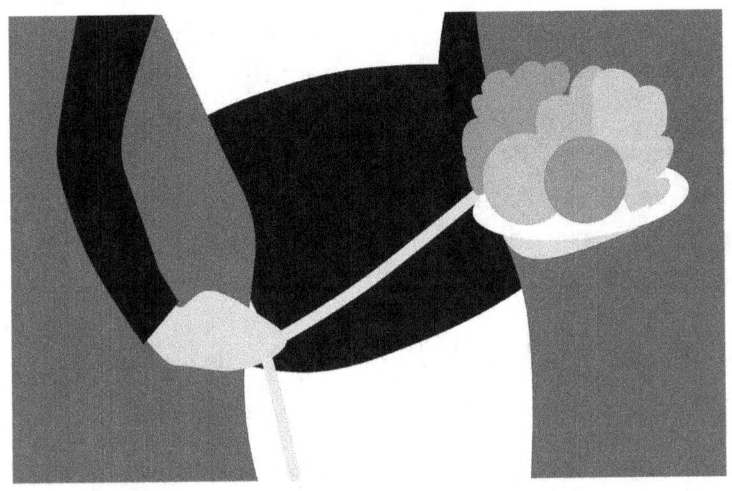

But what did that mean? It meant shedding excess weight, feeling more energetic, and building a healthier relationship with my body. This defined goal became the cornerstone of my daily motivation.

3. Breaking Down the Goal

A broad goal like "burn fat" needed breaking down into manageable parts. This challenge was a blend of various exercises – from high-intensity cardio to bodyweight strength training. Each day had a specific focus, targeting different muscle groups and keeping the routine dynamic. This structure prevented monotony and kept me engaged.

4. The No-Equipment Advantage

One of the beauties of this challenge was its accessibility. Gym membership and costly equipment are not needed. The workouts were designed to utilize the body's weight – simple yet effective. Squats, lunges, planks – these became my companions, and they required nothing more than commitment and consistency.

Jumping Jacks: A full-body cardio exercise to kickstart the heart rate.

Bodyweight Squats: Engaging the lower body for strength and endurance.

Mountain Climbers: Working the core and improving cardiovascular health.

These exercises formed the backbone of my daily routine, and their simplicity made the challenge feasible for beginners like me.

5. The Role of Consistency

Consistency is the silent force behind any fitness journey. As the days progressed, I realized the power of showing up every day. Some days were challenging – fatigue, sore muscles – but pushing through became a testament to my commitment. It was a gradual metamorphosis, and the small wins along the way kept me going.

6. Adapting to Individual Pace

Each person's fitness journey is unique, and this challenge acknowledged that. The exercises were scalable – starting from beginner-friendly variations and gradually progressing. This adaptability ensured that anyone, regardless of their fitness level, could embark on this journey and experience positive changes.

7. The Mental Shift

Beyond the physical transformation, the challenge prompted a shift in mindset. It wasn't just about losing inches; it was about proving to myself that I could stick to something, that change was possible. The daily commitment created a rhythm, a newfound discipline that spilled over into other aspects of my life.

8. Celebrating Progress

Amidst the sweat and effort, celebrating progress was crucial. Whether it was completing more reps, feeling stronger, or noticing subtle changes in my body, these were the victories that fueled my motivation. The scale was only one measure; the real triumphs were in the daily grind.

9. Lessons Learned

As the 30 days concluded, the lessons learned were invaluable. I understood the importance of setting specific goals, the power of consistency, and the adaptability of workouts to individual needs. The challenge was not just a physical endeavor; it was a journey of self-discovery.

10. The Next pop

Understanding your fitness goals isn't a one-time event – it's an ongoing process. This challenge served as a catalyst, propelling me into a world of possibilities. It became a stepping stone to crafting personalized fitness goals and routines tailored to my aspirations.

As we embark on this journey together, remember that your goals are unique to you. Whether it's a 30-day challenge, a marathon, or simply feeling more energetic, define your destination. This chapter is your starting point, a compass to guide you towards a healthier, stronger you. The adventure awaits – let's discover it together.

1.2: ASSESSING YOUR FITNESS LEVEL

Embarking on a fitness journey is like setting sail on a sea of possibilities, and before navigating the waves, it's crucial to chart your course. Assessing your fitness level serves as the compass, guiding you towards a healthier, stronger version of yourself. In this chapter, we'll explore the importance of understanding where you stand on the fitness spectrum and how my personal experience with a "30 Days Fat Burning Challenge for Total Beginners without Equipment" can illuminate this path.

The Starting Line

Imagine standing at the starting line of a race, the anticipation palpable in the air. Your fitness journey begins here. Acknowledging your current state is the first step towards progress. My own journey kick-started with a realization – a desire for change. Reflecting on my sedentary lifestyle, I embarked on a 30-day challenge tailored for beginners with no need for fancy gym equipment.

Setting the Stage

To assess your fitness level, let's break it down into key components:

1. Cardiovascular Endurance

Picture yourself climbing a flight of stairs or briskly walking to catch a bus. These everyday activities involve cardiovascular endurance. In my 30-day challenge, I incorporated activities like brisk walking, jumping jacks, and jogging in place. Gradually, I noticed an increase in my stamina and the ability to tackle these tasks with newfound ease.

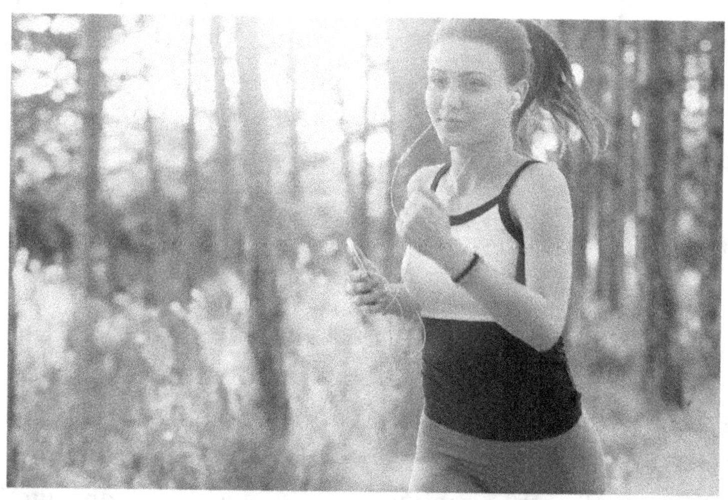

2. Strength and Muscular Endurance

Lifting grocery bags, carrying a toddler, or even opening a tight jar - these scenarios call for strength and muscular endurance. Bodyweight exercises such as squats, push-ups, and lunges became my companions in the challenge. Documenting the gradual improvement in my ability to perform these exercises became a tangible measure of progress.

3. Flexibility

It is often disregarded yet it holds a key position in overall general fitness. Simple stretches and yoga poses were integrated into my routine. The increased flexibility not only enhanced my performance in workouts but also translated into improved posture and reduced muscle tension.

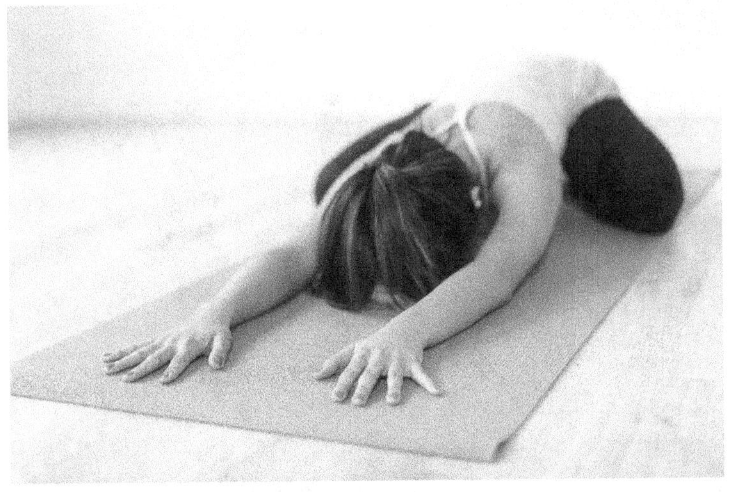

Reflecting on Progress

Consistent self-assessment is the key to any successful journey. In my case, keeping a journal allowed me to track daily activities, note improvements, and identify areas that needed extra attention. This tangible record became a motivational tool, showcasing the progress made over the 30 days.

The Power of Progress Photos

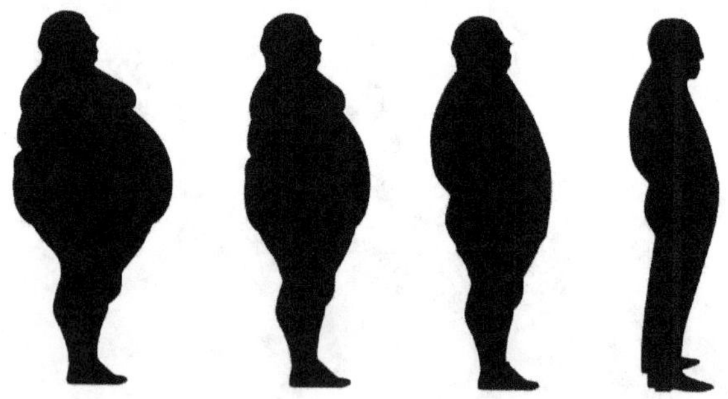

A picture speaks a thousand words, and in the fitness world, progress photos are your visual diary. Documenting my journey through photographs provided a clear visual of the transformation – a powerful motivator on days when enthusiasm waned. I encourage you to capture your own journey, celebrating every small victory.

Understanding Your Body's Feedback

Our bodies communicate, and tuning into these signals is crucial. Throughout my challenge, I learned to listen to my body – acknowledging sore muscles as a sign of growth, understanding fatigue as a call for rest, and recognizing increased energy levels as a reward for consistent effort.

Embracing the Journey

In conclusion, assessing your fitness level is not a one-time event but an ongoing process. My 30-day challenge was a catalyst for change, a personalized roadmap that illuminated the path to a healthier lifestyle. Embrace your journey with curiosity and determination, using self-assessment as your compass, and you'll discover the transformative power of incremental progress.

As we venture into subsequent chapters, we'll delve deeper into specific exercises, nutrition guidance, and mental wellness strategies. Remember, every step forward, no matter how small, is a triumph on your unique fitness expedition.

1.3: SETTING REALISTIC TARGETS

Embarking on a fitness journey without a destination in mind is like setting sail without a map. In this chapter, we'll explore the art of setting realistic targets, an essential compass that ensures your path is both achievable and rewarding. Drawing on my personal experience with a "30 Days Fat Burning Challenge for Total Beginners without Equipment," we'll navigate through the process of establishing goals that propel you toward success.

The Pitfall of Unrealistic Expectations

Imagine starting a journey with the expectation of reaching a distant peak overnight. Unrealistic goals can be demotivating and set the stage for disappointment. My initial foray into fitness taught me the importance of setting targets that are challenging yet attainable. The 30-day challenge became my testing ground for this principle.

Defining Your Starting Point

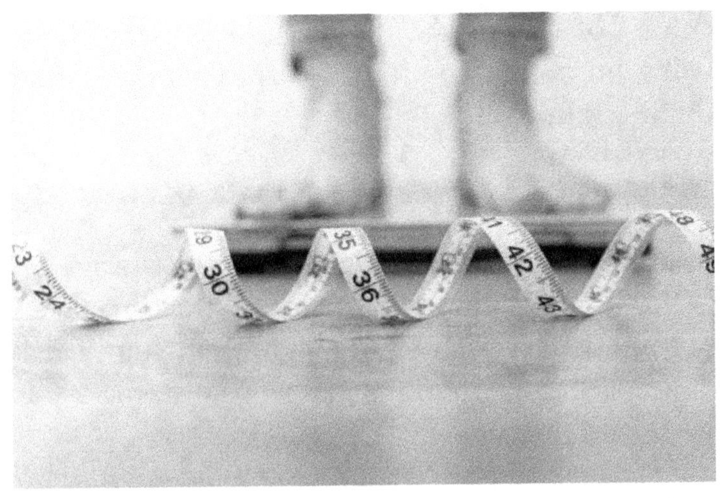

Before outlining your fitness targets, it's crucial to understand your baseline. Reflect on where you currently stand in terms of endurance, strength, and flexibility. My 30-day challenge served as a valuable baseline assessment, revealing areas that needed improvement and strengths waiting to be harnessed.

SMART Goal Setting

The SMART criteria – Specific, Measurable, Achievable, Relevant, and Time-bound – offer a practical framework for goal setting. Let's break it down:

1. Specific

Rather than a vague goal like "lose weight," be specific. In my challenge, I aimed to incorporate 30 minutes of moderate-intensity exercise daily, focusing on a combination of cardio, strength, and flexibility training.

2. Measurable

Tangible metrics provide a clear gauge of progress. Whether it's the number of push-ups, the time taken for a mile run, or the inches lost around your waist, having measurable markers allows you to track your journey with precision.

3. Achievable

Setting goals that are within reach prevents frustration and promotes motivation. My challenge targeted a gradual weight loss of 1-2 pounds per week, a realistic and sustainable pace.

4. Relevant

Align your goals with your overarching objective. If improved cardiovascular health is your aim, incorporate activities like jogging or cycling. My challenge was tailored to burn fat, aligning with my broader goal of overall fitness.

5. Time-bound

Without a time limit, a goal is just a desire. Establishing a timeframe creates a sense of urgency and commitment. My 30-day challenge provided a structured timeline, infusing each day with purpose and accountability.

Tailoring Goals to Your Lifestyle

Life is dynamic, and so should be your fitness goals. Consider your daily schedule, commitments, and preferences. In my experience, crafting goals that seamlessly integrated into my routine increased the likelihood of adherence.

Celebrating Milestones, Big and Small

In the pursuit of larger goals, celebrating milestones is essential. Completing a challenging workout, achieving a personal best, or consistently following your routine for a week – these are victories worth acknowledging. My challenge was punctuated with small celebrations, reinforcing the positive momentum.

Adjusting Course When Necessary

Flexibility is not just for stretching; it's a vital aspect of goal setting. During my 30-day challenge, I encountered days when fatigue set in or unexpected events disrupted my routine. Instead of viewing these as setbacks, I learned to adjust my goals temporarily, maintaining progress in a realistic manner.

The Power of Visualization

One powerful technique for reaching your objectives is visualization.

Envision yourself conquering a challenging workout or reaching a specific fitness milestone. This mental imagery can enhance motivation and drive.

Balancing Ambition and Patience

While ambition fuels progress, patience sustains it. My 30-day challenge taught me that results takes time. Balancing the eagerness for change with the understanding that transformations unfold gradually is a delicate yet crucial aspect of setting realistic targets.

Moving Forward with Purpose

In conclusion, setting realistic targets is the compass that directs your fitness journey. My personal encounter with the 30-day challenge emphasized the importance of aligning goals with your starting point, employing the SMART criteria, tailoring goals to your lifestyle, celebrating milestones, adapting when needed, visualizing success, and maintaining a delicate balance between ambition and patience.

As we proceed to subsequent chapters, we'll delve into refining your workout routine, exploring dietary considerations, and nurturing mental resilience. Remember, each goal achieved, no matter how modest, propels you closer to a healthier, stronger version of yourself. Embrace the process, set your targets wisely, and revel in the journey ahead.

1.4: THE CRUCIAL RITUALS - IMPORTANCE OF WARM-UP AND COOL-DOWN

In the journey of fitness, one often hears about the exhilarating highs of challenging workouts and the triumphant victories of achieving fitness goals. However, nestled between these tales of success lies a chapter often overlooked but integral to any fitness narrative – the importance of warm-ups and cool-downs. In my personal exploration of fitness, particularly during a 30-day Fat Burning Challenge tailored for total beginners without the need for specialized exercise equipment.

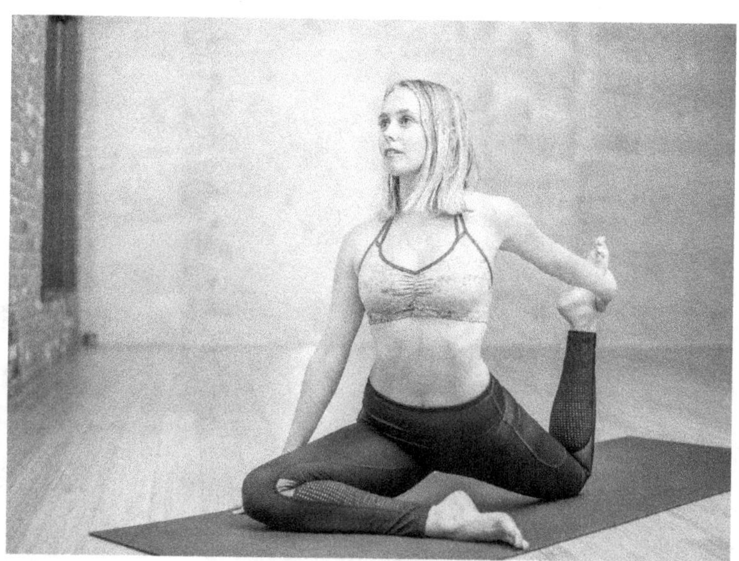

The Prelude: Understanding Warm-ups

Before delving into the heart of my fitness journey, it's crucial to shed light on the significance of warm-ups. Picture this – your body is like an engine, and just as a cold engine struggles to perform optimally, your muscles and joints need a gradual warm-up to kickstart their functions efficiently. Warm-ups serve as the body's gentle wake-up call, preparing it for the upcoming physical demands.

The Physiology of Warm-ups

To grasp the essence of warm-ups, let's peer into the physiology. When you engage in light aerobic activities during a warm-up, your heart rate gradually increases, pumping more blood to the muscles. This increased blood flow enhances the delivery of oxygen and nutrients, priming the muscles for action. Simultaneously, your joints benefit from improved lubrication as the synovial fluid production escalates, ensuring smoother movements.

The Unveiling: My 30-Day Fat Burning Challenge

Embarking on a fitness journey, I committed to a 30-day Fat Burning Challenge tailored for total beginners, without the need for any specialized equipment. The allure of this challenge was not only the promise of shedding excess weight but also the simplicity of incorporating it into my daily routine.

The Warm-up Routine

Each session of my 30-day challenge commenced with a purposeful warm-up. From brisk walking and jumping jacks to dynamic stretches, the warm-up was a vital prelude to the main workout. It not only awakened my dormant muscles but also mentally prepared me for the physical exertion ahead.

The Impact: Feeling the Difference

As the days progressed, I keenly observed the impact of incorporating warm-ups into my routine. Initially skeptical, I soon found that the initial sluggishness gave way to a sense of readiness. The gradual increase in heart rate became a cue for my body to switch gears, signaling that it was time to embrace the ensuing challenge.

The Grand Finale: Cool-downs and Their Significance

Now, as we transition from the vigorous main workout, another crucial chapter unfolds – the cool-down. Often dismissed as an afterthought, cool-downs are the serene closure to an intense exercise session.

Preventing Abrupt Halts

Imagine slamming the brakes on a speeding car – a sudden stop could lead to chaos. Similarly, abrupt cessation of intense physical activity can subject your body to stress and potential injuries. Cool-downs, characterized by gentle exercises and stretches, allow your heart rate to gradually return to its resting state, preventing the abrupt halts that can strain your cardiovascular system.

The Healing Touch

Cool-downs also provide a healing touch to your muscles. Engaging in static stretches during this phase helps in reducing muscle tension and preventing the dreaded post-exercise stiffness. As I concluded each session of my 30-day challenge with a deliberate cool-down, I experienced a sense of tranquility, knowing that I was nurturing my body even in the aftermath of intense exertion.

The Continuous Thread: Consistency in Warm-ups and Cool-downs

As my 30-day Fat Burning Challenge progressed, the interplay between warm-ups and cool-downs emerged as a continuous thread weaving through my fitness journey. Consistency in these rituals not only became a source of physical well-being but also a testament to the holistic approach required for sustainable fitness.

Building Habits for a Lifetime

Incorporating warm-ups and cool-downs into my daily routine became second nature. The once underestimated rituals transformed into habits that extended beyond the confines of the 30-day challenge. I realized that the journey to fitness is not a sprint but a marathon, where the mindful inclusion of these rituals lays the foundation for a resilient and enduring commitment to one's well-being.

Conclusion: The Symphony of Fitness

In the grand symphony of fitness, warm-ups and cool-downs compose the overture and finale, respectively. My 30-day Fat Burning Challenge for total beginners without equipment became not just a personal triumph but a testament to the transformative power of these seemingly simple yet profoundly impactful rituals.

As you embark on your own fitness odyssey, remember that the magic lies not just in the intensity of your workout but in the mindful orchestration of the entire symphony. The gentle crescendo of warm-ups prepares the stage, the vigorous main workout takes center stage, and the serene decrescendo of cool-downs concludes the performance, leaving you with a sense of accomplishment and a body ready for the encore of the next challenge.

1.5: SAFETY CONSIDERATIONS , INJURIES and PREVENTION

Safety Considerations, Injury Prevention, and Practical Tips for the 30-Day Fat Burning Challenge for Total Beginners

When embarking on a fitness journey, safety should be your top priority. Whether you're a seasoned fitness enthusiast or a total beginner, understanding safety considerations and injury prevention is crucial. In this chapter, we'll delve into practical tips specifically tailored for total beginners participating in a 30-day fat burning challenge with no equipment. Let's keep it simple, straightforward, and accessible to all.

Safety First: A Fundamental Approach

See a medical expert before beginning any fitness program, particularly if you have any underlying medical issues. Safety starts with understanding your own body and its limitations. Pay attention to your body's signals and move at a speed that suits you.

1. Warm-Up Essentials:

- Begin each session with a 5-10 minute warm-up to prepare your muscles and joints.

- Incorporate light cardio activities like marching in place or jumping jacks to increase blood flow

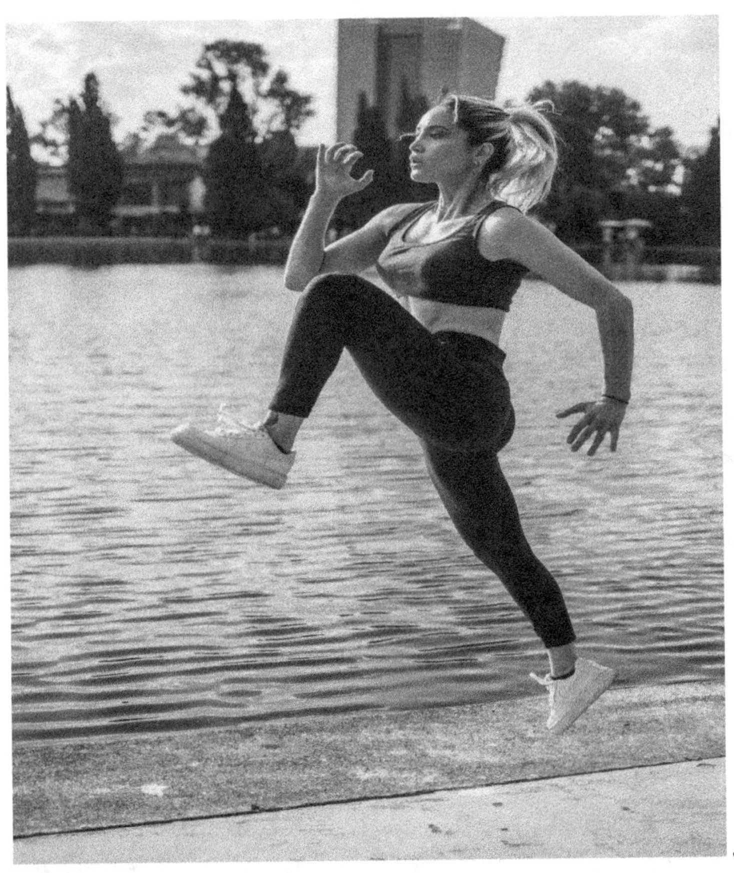

2. Low-Impact Exercises:

- Opt for low-impact exercises to reduce stress on joints and minimize the risk of injuries.

- Examples include brisk walking, cycling, or modified jumping jacks.

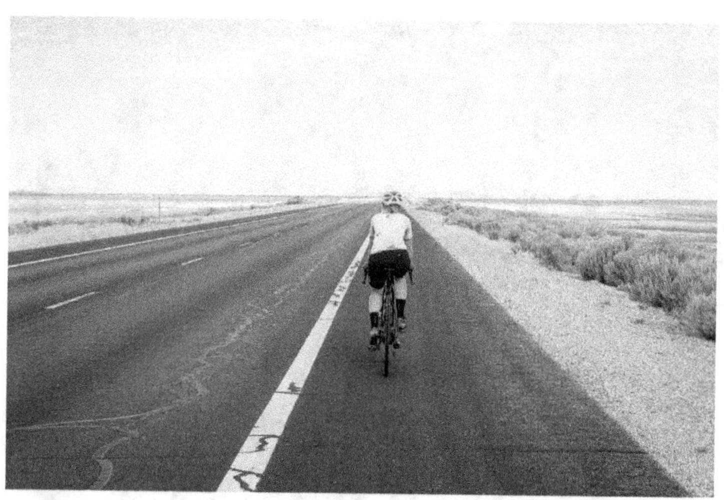

3. Proper Form Over Intensity:

- Focus on mastering proper form before increasing the intensity of your workouts.

- Incorrect form can lead to injuries, so pay attention to your body positioning during exercises.

Understanding Common Injuries and Prevention Strategies

Let's address common concerns and provide practical tips to prevent injuries during your 30-day fat burning challenge.

1. Strains and Sprains:

-Prevention:

Gradually increase exercise intensity, and avoid sudden, forceful movements.

- Tip:

Include dynamic stretching in your warm-up to improve flexibility and reduce strain.

2. Overuse Injuries:

- Prevention:

Rotate exercise routines to avoid repetitive stress on specific muscles or joints.

- Tip:

Your schedule should include rest days so that your body can recuperate.

3. Joint Pain:

- Prevention:

Choose exercises with low impact and incorporate joint-friendly activities.

- Tip:

If you experience persistent joint pain, consult a fitness professional or healthcare provider.

4. Dehydration and Fatigue:

- Prevention:

Stay hydrated throughout the day, and ensure a balanced diet for sustained energy.

- Tip:

Listen to your body; if you feel fatigued, take a break and resume when you're ready.

Practical Tips for the 30-Day Fat Burning Challenge

Now, let's explore practical tips to make your fat burning challenge enjoyable and effective, even as a total beginner with no equipment.

1. Create a Realistic Schedule:

- Set achievable workout goals that fit your daily routine.

- Strive to achieve at least 30 minutes of exercise on the majority of days in a week.

2. Mix Up Your Workouts:

- To target different muscle groups, incorporate a variety of exercises.

- This prevents monotony and engages your body in new ways.

3. Bodyweight Exercises:

- Focus on exercises that use your body weight for resistance.

- Planks, push-ups, squats, and lunges are great options.

4. Interval Training:

- Incorporate short bursts of high-intensity exercises followed by periods of rest.

- This approach boosts metabolism and enhances fat burning.

5. Rest and Recovery:

- Make sure to incorporate rest days to give your muscles the opportunity to recover.

- Adequate sleep is crucial for overall recovery and optimal performance.

6. Nutrition Support:

- Maintain a balanced diet with emphasis on lean proteins, whole grains, and plenty of fruits and vegetables.

- Maintain proper hydration to help your body meet its energy requirements.

7. Tracking Progress:

- Keep a simple journal to track your workouts and how you feel.

- Celebrate small achievements along the way.

8. Mindful Movement:

- Focus on the joy of movement rather than fixating on weight loss.

- Mindful exercise promotes a positive relationship with fitness.

Conclusion: Empowerment Through Safe and Effective Exercise

As you embark on your 30-day fat burning challenge, remember that safety, consistency, and enjoyment are key. By understanding safety considerations, preventing injuries, and implementing practical tips, you're setting yourself up for a successful and sustainable fitness journey. Whether you're a total beginner or someone returning to exercise, embrace the process, and let each day be a step towards a healthier, fitter you.

CHAPTER 2: BASIC BEGINNERS NUTRITION TIPS FOR ENHANCED RESULTS

2.1: UNDERSTANDING MACRONUTRIENT .

In the realm of fitness, what you eat plays a crucial role in achieving your goals. Understanding macronutrients—proteins, fats, and carbohydrates—is fundamental to fueling your body effectively during a 30-day fat burning challenge. Let's break down these macronutrients in a straightforward manner and provide practical tips for total beginners with no equipment.

Macronutrient Basics: Fueling Your Body Right

1. Proteins: The Building Blocks

- What They Do: Proteins are essential for building and repairing tissues, including muscles.

- Practical Tip: Include lean protein sources like chicken, fish, beans, and tofu in your meals to support muscle health during your challenge.

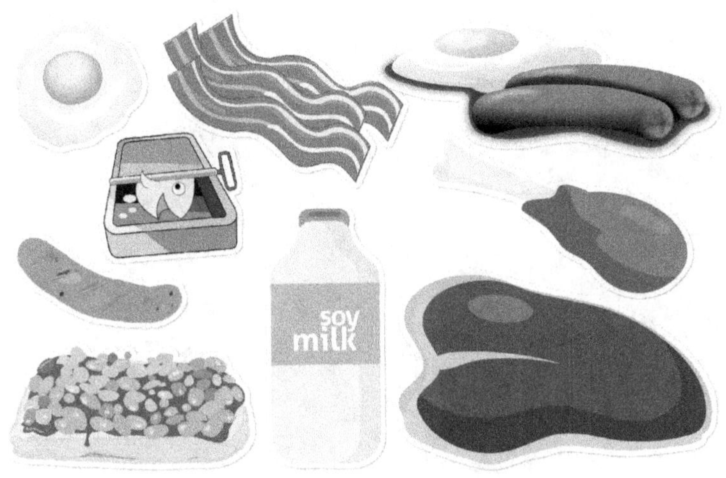

2. Fats: A Source of Energy

- What They Do: Fats provide sustained energy and support various bodily functions.

- Practical Tip: Choose healthy fats found in avocados, nuts, seeds, and olive oil to keep you energized throughout your workouts.

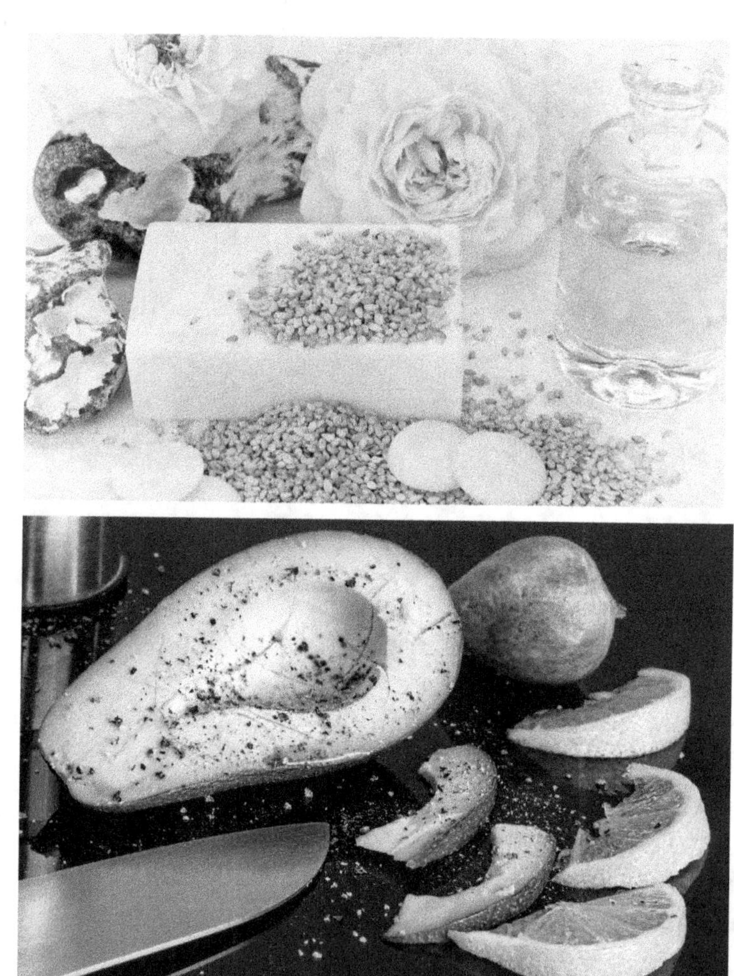

3. Carbohydrates: Your Body's Preferred Fuel

- What They Do: Carbs are the primary energy source for your body, especially during exercise.

- Practical Tip: Prioritize complex carbohydrates such as whole grains, fruits, and vegetables for sustained energy and overall health.

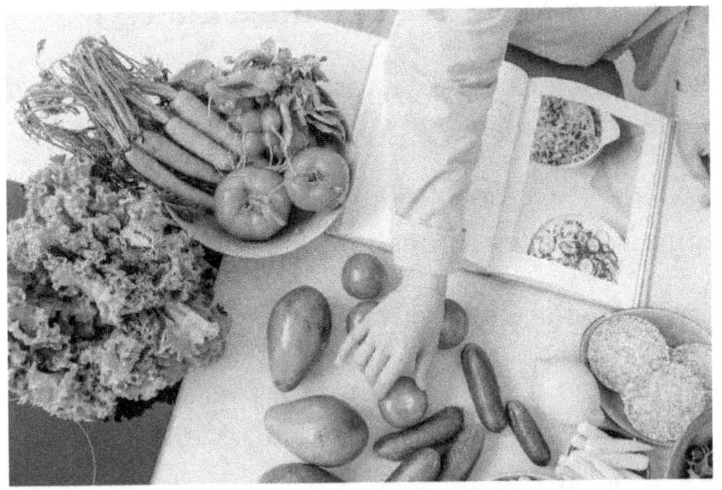

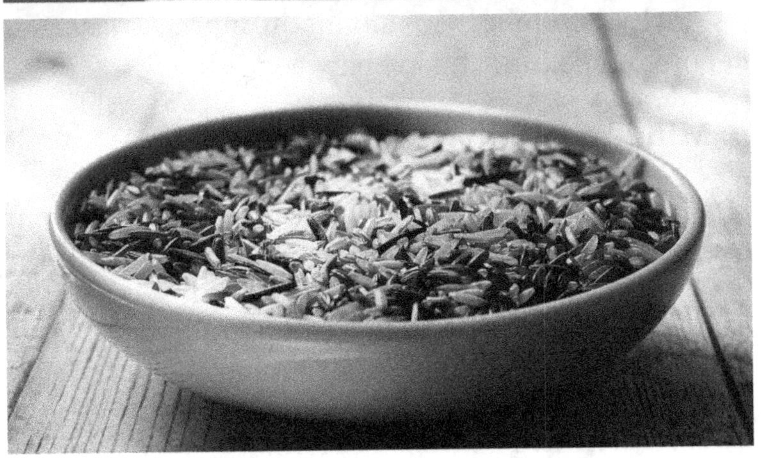

Practical Tips for Your 30-Day Fat Burning Challenge:

1. Balanced Meals for Sustained Energy:

   - Tip: Aim for balanced meals that include a mix of proteins, fats, and carbohydrates.

   - Why: This provides a steady release of energy, keeping you fueled throughout the day.

2. Protein-Packed Snacks:

   - Tip: Incorporate protein-rich snacks like Greek yogurt, cottage cheese, or a handful of nuts.

   - Why: Protein helps maintain muscle mass and keeps you feeling satisfied between meals.

3. Mindful Portion Control:

   - Tip: Pay attention to portion sizes to prevent overindulging.

   - Why: Understanding portion control supports your overall calorie balance for fat burning.

4. Hydration: The Unsung Hero:

- Tip: Drink an adequate amount of water throughout the day.

- Why: Staying hydrated is crucial for overall health and supports optimal metabolic function.

5. Pre-Workout Fuel:

- Tip: Consume a light meal or snack containing carbohydrates and a small amount of protein before your workout.

- Why: This provides the energy needed for an effective workout.

6. Post-Workout Recovery:

- Tip: Include a source of protein in your post-workout meal or snack.

- Why: Protein aids muscle recovery and helps replenish energy stores.

7. Whole Foods vs. Processed Foods:

- Tip: Choose whole, unprocessed foods over highly processed options.

- Why: Whole foods provide more nutrients and contribute to overall well-being.

8. Healthy Fats for Satiety:

- Tip: Include sources of healthy fats in your meals to enhance satiety.

- Why: Healthy fats contribute to a feeling of fullness and satisfaction.

Navigating Macronutrients in Your Daily Meals:

Breakfast:

- Include whole-grain oats for complex carbs.

- Add Greek yogurt or eggs for protein.

- Top with fruits for natural sweetness and additional nutrients.

Lunch:

- Opt for a lean protein source such as grilled chicken or beans.

- Include a variety of colorful vegetables.

- Go for dressings with olive oil for a healthy fat choice.

Dinner:

- Incorporate fish or tofu for protein.

- Include a mix of leafy greens and other veggies.

- Use quinoa or brown rice for complex carbs.

Snacks:

- Pair apple slices with almond butter for a balance of carbs and healthy fats.

- Snack on a handful of mixed nuts for a quick protein boost.

- Greek yogurt with berries makes for a protein-packed and refreshing snack.

Conclusion: Fueling Your Success

Understanding macronutrients doesn't have to be complicated. By incorporating a variety of whole foods and being mindful of your protein, fat, and carbohydrate intake, you'll be well-fueled for your 30-day fat burning challenge. Practical tips like balanced meals, proper hydration, and mindful portion control can make a significant difference in your energy levels and overall well-being. Keep it simple, enjoy your meals, and let the right fuel propel you toward success in your fitness journey.

2.2: HYDRATION FOR OPTIMAL PERFORMANCE

Hydration is a game-changer when it comes to your fitness journey. In this chapter, we'll break down the importance of staying well-hydrated during your 30-day fat burning challenge. Let's keep it simple, straightforward, and packed with practical tips for total beginners with no equipment.

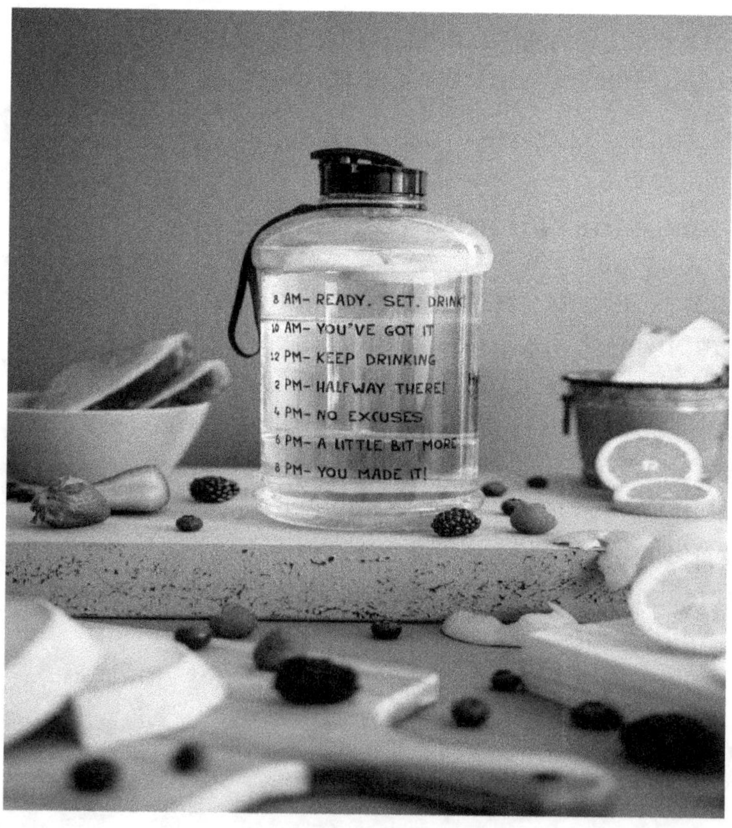

The Basics: Why Hydration Matters

1. Optimal Performance:

- Why It Matters: Proper hydration ensures your body functions at its best during workouts.

- Practical Tip: Aim to drink water consistently throughout the day, not just during exercise.

2. Temperature Regulation:

- Why It Matters: Sweating is your body's natural cooling mechanism, and staying hydrated supports this process.

- Practical Tip: Pay attention to your body's signals — if you're sweating, make sure you're replenishing fluids.

3. Energy Levels:

- Why It Matters: Dehydration can lead to fatigue and decreased energy levels.

- Practical Tip: Drink water regularly to maintain steady energy throughout the day.

4. Muscle Function:

- Why It Matters: Well-hydrated muscles are more efficient and less prone to cramping.

- Practical Tip: Hydrate before, during, and after your workouts to support muscle function.

Practical Hydration Tips for Your 30-Day Challenge:

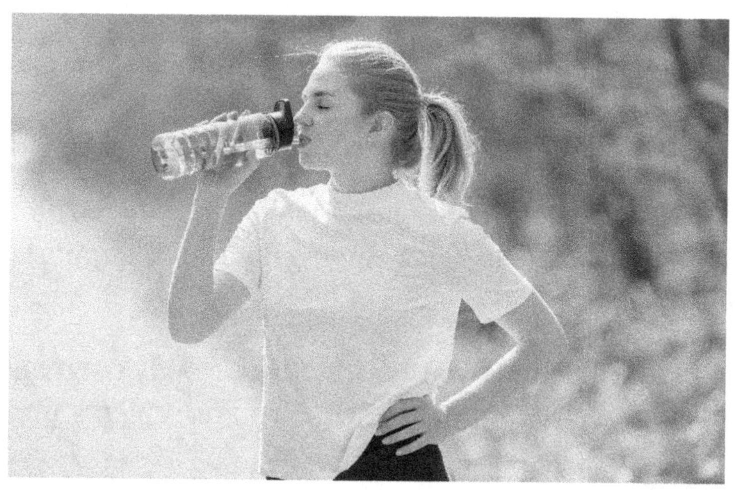

1. Consistent sipping throughout the day:

- Tip: Keep a water bottle within reach and take sips consistently.

- Why: This helps maintain hydration levels and prevents the need to chug large amounts at once.

2. Set a hydration goal:

   - Tip: Aim for at least 8 cups (64 ounces) of water per day, adjusting based on your activity level and climate.

   - Why: Having a goal gives you a tangible target to ensure adequate hydration.

3. Infuse with flavor:

   - Tip: Add natural flavors like cucumber, lemon, or mint to your water.

   - Why: Infused water can make hydration more enjoyable, encouraging you to drink more.

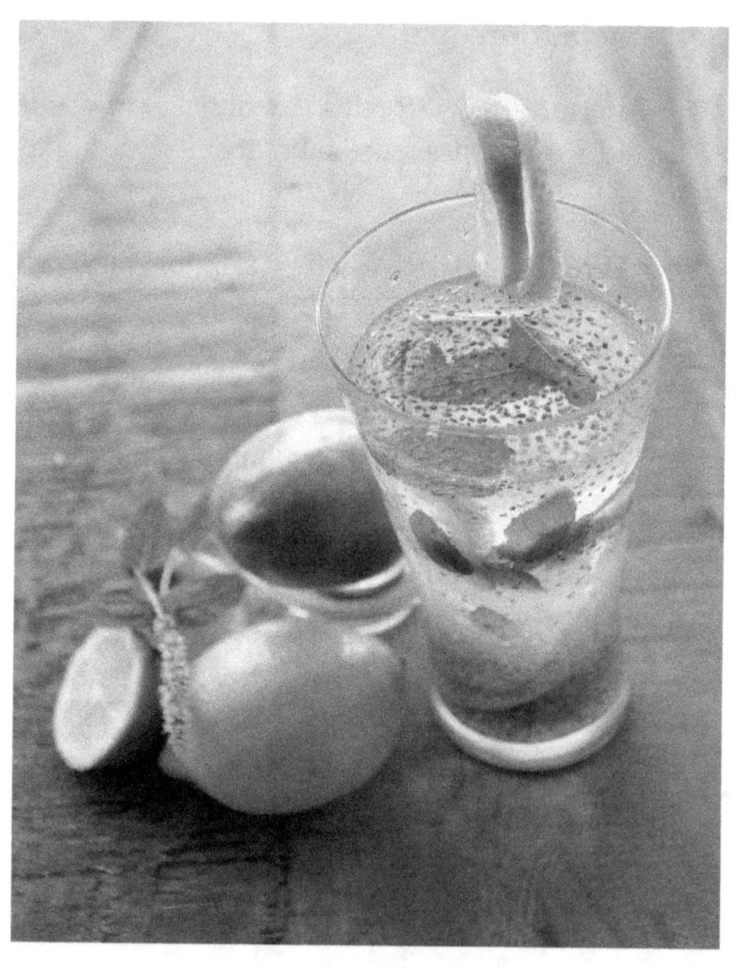

4. Track your intake:

- Tip: Use a water tracking app or a simple journal to monitor your daily water intake.

- Why: Tracking helps you stay accountable and ensures you meet your hydration goals.

5. Hydrate before meals:

- Tip: Drink a glass of water before each meal.

- Why: This not only supports hydration but can also help control appetite during your fat-burning challenge.

6. Include hydrating foods:

- Tip: Consume water-rich foods like watermelon, cucumber, and oranges.

- Why: These foods contribute to your overall fluid intake and provide additional nutrients.

7. Monitor urine color:

- Tip: Check the color of your urine – pale yellow is a good indicator of proper hydration.

- Why: Dark yellow urine may signal dehydration, while clear urine might suggest overhydration.

8. Hydrate during exercise:

- Tip: Ensure to stay hydrated by consuming water before, during, and after your workout sessions.

- Why: Hydrating during exercise is crucial to replace fluids lost through sweat.

Navigating Hydration During Your 30-Day Challenge:

Morning Routine:

-Drink a glass of water first thing in the morning to stay hydrated.

- Consider a cup of herbal tea for added hydration and antioxidants.

Pre-Workout Hydration:

- Consume water about 1-2 hours before your workout.

- For early morning workouts, hydrate as soon as you wake up.

During Exercise:

- Take small sips of water during your workout, especially if it's intense.

- Consider water-rich snacks like slices of cucumber or watermelon.

Post-Workout Recovery:

- Rehydrate with water after your workout to replenish fluid losses.

- Include a source of electrolytes if your workout was particularly intense.

Evening Routine:

- Wind down with a cup of herbal tea or warm water.

- Avoid excessive caffeine or sugary beverages close to bedtime.

Conclusion: Stay Refreshed, Stay Energized

Staying hydrated is a simple yet powerful component of your 30-day fat burning challenge. By adopting practical tips like consistent sipping, setting hydration goals, and including water-rich foods, you'll be supporting optimal performance, energy levels, and muscle function. Keep it straightforward, make hydration a habit, and let the refreshing benefits propel you towards success in your fitness journey.

2.3: THE CRUCIAL ROLE OF WHOLE FOODS

In this chapter, we'll delve into the importance of whole foods in fueling your body during a 30-day fat burning challenge. Let's keep it clear, simple, and loaded with practical tips for total beginners without any equipment.

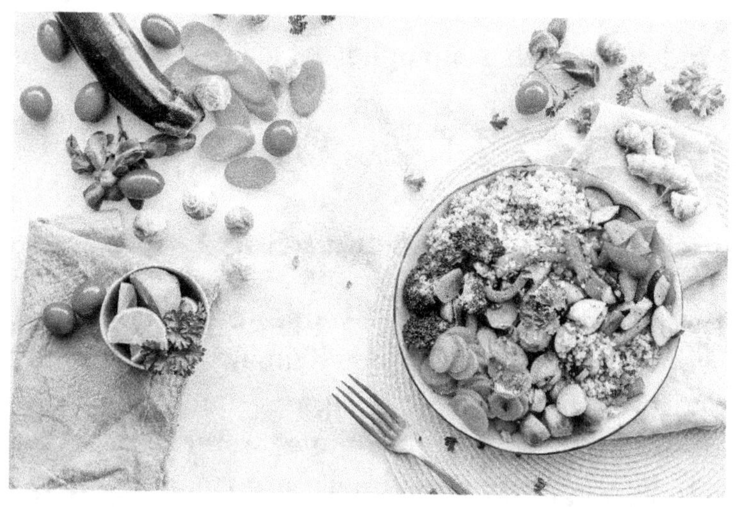

Why Whole Foods Matter: The Basics

1. Nutrient Density:

- Why It Matters: Whole foods pack a nutritional punch, offering essential vitamins, minerals, and antioxidants.

- Practical Tip: Prioritize colorful fruits and vegetables to ensure a variety of nutrients.

2. Sustained Energy:

- Why It Matters: Whole foods, such as complex carbohydrates, provide a steady release of energy.

- Practical Tip: Opt for whole grains like brown rice, quinoa, and oats to fuel your workouts.

3. Fiber for Satiety:

- Why It Matters: Fiber-rich foods keep you feeling full, supporting appetite control.

- Practical Tip: Include sources of fiber like beans, lentils, and vegetables in your meals.

4. Lean Protein Sources:

- Why It Matters: Protein is crucial for muscle repair and maintenance, especially during a fat burning challenge.

- Practical Tip: Choose lean protein sources such as chicken, fish, tofu, and legumes.

5. Micronutrient Support:

   - Why It Matters: Whole foods provide a spectrum of micronutrients essential for overall health.

   - Practical Tip: Incorporate a variety of fruits and vegetables to cover a range of vitamins and minerals.

Practical Tips for Including Whole Foods:

1. Build Balanced Meals:

   - Tip: Include a mix of protein, carbohydrates, and healthy fats in each meal.

   - Why: Balanced meals provide a range of nutrients for overall health and energy.

2. Choose Colorful Produce:

   - Tip: Aim to fill half your plate with colorful fruits and vegetables.

   - Why:Different colors signify various nutrients, contributing to a well-rounded diet.

3. Limit Processed Foods:

   - Tip: Minimize the intake of processed foods high in added sugars and unhealthy fats.

- Why: Whole foods are nutrient-dense and provide more health benefits than processed options.

4. Prepare Simple Whole Snacks:

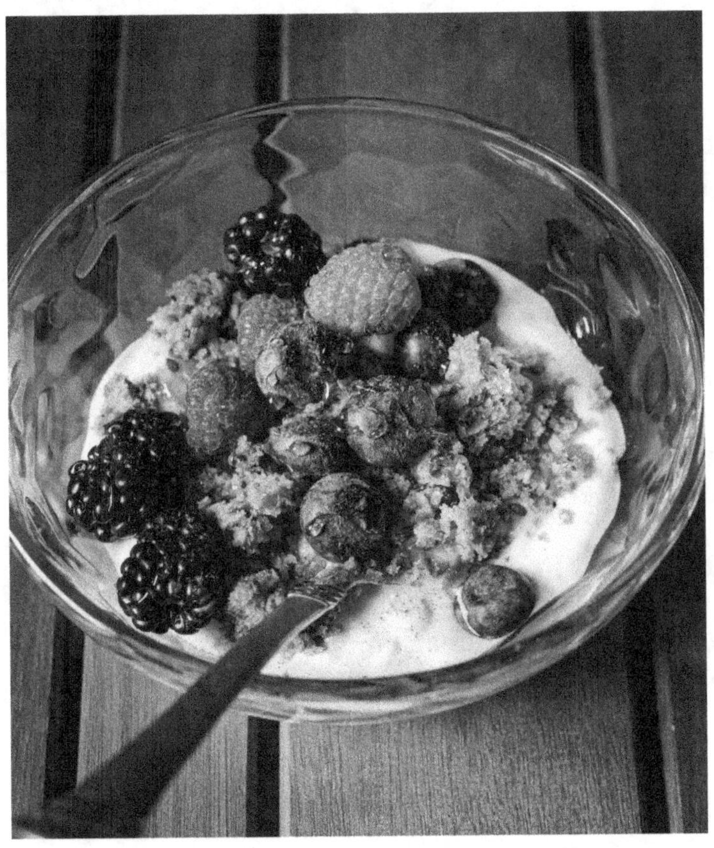

- Tip: Snack on whole foods like apple slices with nut butter, Greek yogurt, or a handful of nuts.

- Why: Whole snacks contribute to sustained energy and keep you satisfied between meals.

5. Incorporate Whole Grains:

- Tip:Choose whole grains like brown rice, quinoa, and whole wheat over refined grains.

- Why: Whole grains offer more fiber and nutrients, aiding in digestion and providing lasting energy.

6. Mindful Eating Habits:

- Tip: Eat slowly, savoring each bite, and pay attention to hunger and fullness cues.

- Why: Mindful eating promotes better digestion and helps prevent overeating.

7. Plan and Prep Ahead:

- Tip: Plan your meals and snacks in advance and prep ingredients for easy access.

- Why: This reduces the temptation to opt for convenience foods and ensures healthier choices.

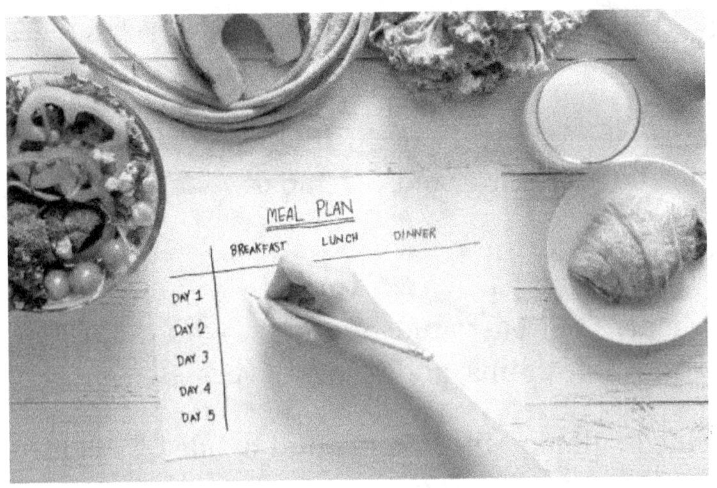

8. Stay Hydrated with Whole Beverages:

- Tip: Choose water, herbal tea, or infused water over sugary beverages.

- Why: Hydrating with whole beverages supports overall health without added sugars.

Navigating Whole Foods in Your Daily Routine:

Breakfast:

- Opt for a whole-food-rich breakfast like oatmeal topped with berries and nuts.

- Include a protein source like Greek yogurt or eggs.

Lunch:

- Build a balanced lunch with a variety of vegetables, lean protein, and whole grains.

- Consider a colorful salad with grilled chicken or a quinoa bowl with roasted vegetables.

Dinner:

- Prepare a well-rounded dinner with a protein source, whole grains, and plenty of veggies.

- Grilled salmon with quinoa and a side of steamed broccoli is a nutritious option.

Snacks:

- Snack on whole fruits, such as apple slices or a banana.

- Consider vegetable sticks with hummus or a small handful of nuts for a satisfying snack.

Conclusion: Fueling Success with Whole Foods

As you embark on your 30-day fat burning challenge, remember that whole foods are your allies in achieving sustainable and healthy results. By incorporating practical tips like building balanced meals, choosing colorful produce, and limiting processed foods, you're not just nourishing your body but also enhancing your overall well-being. Keep it simple, enjoy the variety of whole foods available, and let the natural goodness propel you towards success in your fitness journey

2.4: PRE -and POST-WORKOUT NUTRITION

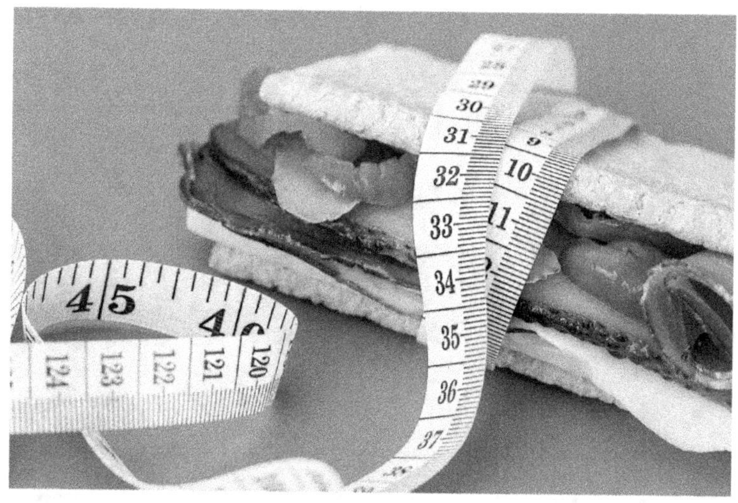

Fueling your body effectively before and after workouts is paramount in maximizing the benefits of your 30-day fat burning challenge. In this chapter, we'll keep it simple and provide practical tips for total beginners without any equipment.

Pre-Workout Nutrition: Energizing Your Exercise

1. Timing Matters:

   - When to Eat: Consume a balanced meal or snack 1-2 hours before exercising.

   - Why: Pre-workout nutrition provides the energy needed for a productive workout.

2. Balanced Macros:

   - What to Eat: Include a mix of carbohydrates, protein, and a small amount of healthy fats.

   - *lWhy: Carbs provide immediate energy, protein supports muscle function, and fats aid in sustained energy.

3. Hydration is Key:

   - What to Drink: Drink water consistently leading up to your workout.

   - Why:Proper hydration supports overall performance and prevents dehydration during exercise.

4. Pre-Workout Snack Ideas:

   - Option 1: Greek yogurt with berries and a sprinkle of granola.

- Option 2: Whole grain toast with nut butter and banana slices.

- Option 3: A small smoothie with spinach, fruit, and protein powder.

Practical Tips for Pre-Workout Nutrition:

1. Listen to Your Body:

- Tip: Pay attention to how different foods make you feel before exercise.

- Why: Understanding your body's response helps tailor pre-workout choices.

2. Avoid Heavy Meals:

- Tip: Opt for easily digestible meals or snacks.

- Why: Heavy meals can lead to discomfort during workouts; lighter options are better tolerated.

3. Experiment with Timing:

- Tip: Find the timing that works best for you—some may prefer a larger meal 2 hours before, while others may opt for a smaller snack 30-60 minutes before.

- Why: Personal preferences and digestive differences play a role in optimal timing.

Post-Workout Nutrition: Supporting Recovery

1. Timing Matters (Again):

- When to Eat: Consume a post-workout meal or snack within 30 minutes to an hour after exercising.

- Why: This window is crucial for replenishing glycogen stores and aiding muscle recovery.

2. Protein for Repair:

- What to Eat: Prioritize a protein source along with carbohydrates.

- Why: Protein supports muscle repair and growth, while carbs replenish energy stores.

3. Hydration Continues:

- What to Drink: Continue hydrating with water.

- Why: Hydration aids in the recovery process and helps prevent dehydration post-exercise.

4. Post-Workout Snack Ideas:

   - Option 1: Chocolate milk (providing protein and carbs).

   - Option 2: A turkey or chicken sandwich on whole grain bread.

   - Option 3: A smoothie with protein powder, fruits, and yogurt.

Practical Tips for Post-Workout Nutrition:

1. Don't Skip Meals:

   - Tip: Even if your workout is not during a traditional mealtime, ensure you have a post-workout snack.

   - Why: Consistent nutrition supports recovery and overall energy levels.

2. Tailor to Your Goals:

   -Tip: Adjust post-workout nutrition based on your fitness goals.

   - Why: Whether it's weight loss or muscle gain, adapting your nutrient intake supports specific objectives.

3. Whole Food Options:

   - Tip: While shakes or bars are convenient, whole food options are equally effective.

   - Why: Whole foods provide additional nutrients and can be satisfying and enjoyable.

4. Stay Consistent:

  - Tip: Develop a routine for post-workout nutrition.

   - Why: Consistency reinforces healthy habits and aids in overall progress.

Navigating Nutrition Throughout the Day:

Morning Routine:

- Pre-Workout: A banana with a small handful of nuts.

- Post-Workout: Greek yogurt with honey and a sprinkle of granola.

Lunch:

- Pre-Workout (if in the afternoon): Whole grain wrap with turkey, veggies, and hummus.

- Post-Workout: Grilled chicken salad with quinoa and a variety of colorful vegetables.

Dinner:

- Pre-Workout (if in the evening): Baked sweet potato with a side of steamed broccoli.

- Post-Workout: Baked salmon with quinoa and roasted Brussels sprouts.

Snacks:

- Pre-Workout: Whole grain crackers with cheese.

- Post-Workout: Cottage cheese with pineapple chunks.

Conclusion: Fueling Your Success, One Bite at a Time

Optimizing your pre- and post-workout nutrition is a tangible way to enhance your 30-day fat burning challenge. By keeping it simple—balancing macros, staying hydrated, and choosing whole foods—you're providing your body with the support it needs for optimal performance and recovery. Whether you're a morning exerciser or prefer an evening workout, tailor your nutrition to fit your routine and goals. Consistency is key.

2.5: THE ART OF LISTENING TO YOUR BODY

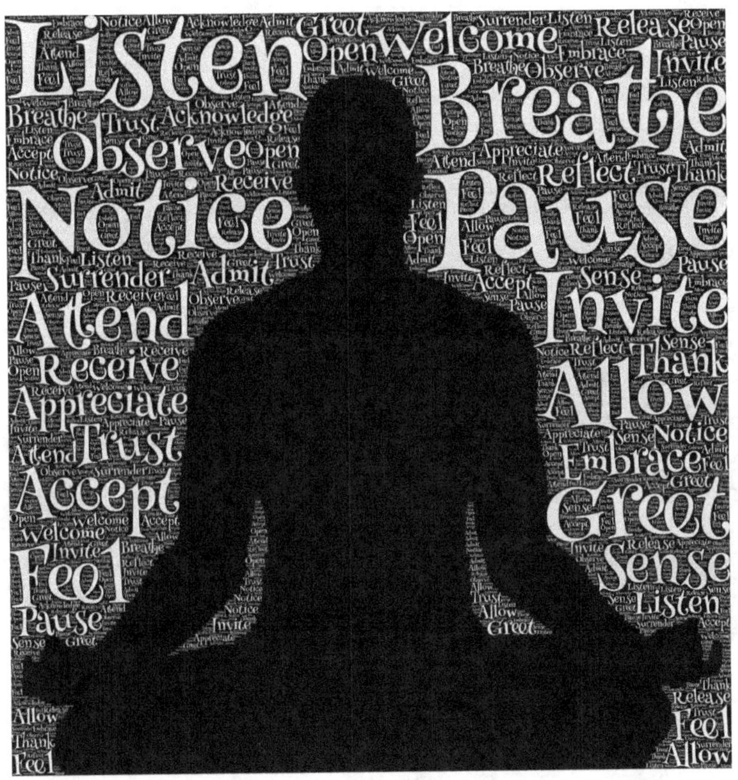

In the journey to a healthier you, one of the most essential skills you can develop is listening to your body. In this chapter, we'll explore the significance of tuning in to your body's signals during a 30-day fat burning challenge. Let's keep it straightforward and provide practical tips for total beginners without any equipment.

Understanding Your Body's Language

1. Recognizing Physical Cues:

   - What to Look For: Pay attention to sensations like hunger, fullness, fatigue, and soreness.

   - Practical Tip: Keep a journal to track how your body responds to different foods and exercises.

2. Distinguishing Between Discomfort and Pain:

   - How to Differentiate: Discomfort is a natural part of exercising, but pain may indicate an issue.

   - Practical Tip: If an exercise causes sharp or persistent pain, modify or consult a fitness professional.

3. Noticing Energy Levels:

   - Signs of Energy: Feeling energized during and after workouts.

   - Practical Tip: Adjust your exercise intensity based on your energy levels on a given day.

4. Acknowledging Emotional Well-Being:

- Connection to Exercise: Note how exercise impacts your mood and stress levels.

- Practical Tip: Engage in activities that bring joy, as positive emotions contribute to overall well-being.

Practical Tips for Listening to Your Body:

1. Set Realistic Goals:

- Tip: Establish achievable goals based on your current fitness level.

- Why: Realistic goals set the foundation for a positive and sustainable fitness journey.

2. Know Your Limits:

- Tip: Understand your physical limitations and be mindful of pushing too hard.

- Why: Respectful training prevents injuries and fosters a healthier relationship with exercise.

3. Rest and Recovery:

- Tip: Incorporate rest days into your routine to allow your body to recover.

- Why: Rest is essential for muscle repair, preventing burnout, and sustaining long-term motivation.

4. Adapt Workouts as Needed:

- Tip: Modify exercises to suit your comfort and ability level.

- Why: Adjusting workouts prevents strain and fosters a positive exercise experience.

5. Hydrate Wisely:

- Tip: Pay attention to your thirst and hydration needs.

- Why: Proper hydration supports overall performance and prevents dehydration-related issues.

6. Prioritize Sleep:

- Tip: Aim for 7-9 hours of quality sleep each night.

- Why: Sleep is vital for recovery, mood regulation, and overall well-being.

7. Listen to Hunger and Fullness:

- Tip: Eat when you're hungry and stop when you're satisfied.

- Why: Tuning in to hunger and fullness cues supports a balanced and sustainable approach to nutrition.

8. Mindful Movement:

- Tip: Engage in exercises you genuinely enjoy.

- Why: Enjoyable activities promote consistent participation and a positive mindset.

Navigating Your Body's Signals Throughout the Challenge:

Morning Routine:

- Pay attention to how your body feels upon waking — any areas of stiffness or soreness.

- Adjust your workout intensity based on how well-rested and energized you feel.

Pre-Workout:

- Evaluate your energy levels — if fatigued, consider a lighter workout or focus on low-intensity activities.

- Notice how different foods impact your body before exercise; choose options that provide sustained energy.

During Exercise:

- Listen to your breathing and adjust intensity accordingly.

- If an exercise causes discomfort beyond the norm, modify or switch to an alternative.

Post-Workout:

- Take note of how your body responds after exercise – feelings of invigoration or excessive fatigue.

- Refuel with a post-workout snack or meal that aligns with your hunger cues.

Evening Routine:

- Assess your overall stress levels – if high, consider activities like gentle stretching or relaxation exercises.

- Prioritize a good night's sleep and adjust your evening routine to support quality rest.

Conclusion: Empowerment Through Body Awareness

Listening to your body is a powerful tool in navigating your 30-day fat burning challenge. By recognizing physical cues, setting realistic goals, and adapting workouts as needed, you empower yourself to build a sustainable and enjoyable fitness routine. Keep it simple, be kind to your body, and let the art of listening guide you towards success in your journey to a healthier and fitter you.

CHAPTER 3

3.1: WORKOUT FOR SPECIFIC GOALS -BUILDING STRENGTH : A Comprehensive Guide

When embarking on a fitness journey, tailoring your workouts to specific goals is crucial. In this chapter, we delve into the realm of building strength – a fundamental aspect of overall fitness. This comprehensive guide will equip you with the knowledge and practical insights needed to sculpt a stronger, more resilient body.

Understanding the Importance of Strength Training

Strength training isn't just for bodybuilders; it's an essential component for anyone seeking holistic fitness. It enhances muscle tone, boosts metabolism, and fortifies bones. My own journey began with a "30 Days Fat Burning Challenge," a transformative experience designed for total beginners without the need for exercise equipment. The results were not just physical but also mental, underscoring the power of strength training for individuals of all fitness levels.

The Basics: Form and Technique

Before delving into specific exercises, it's crucial to grasp the basics of form and technique. Whether you're performing a squat or a push-up, executing each movement with precision ensures optimal results while minimizing the risk of injury. Let's break down a few foundational exercises:

1. Bodyweight Squats:

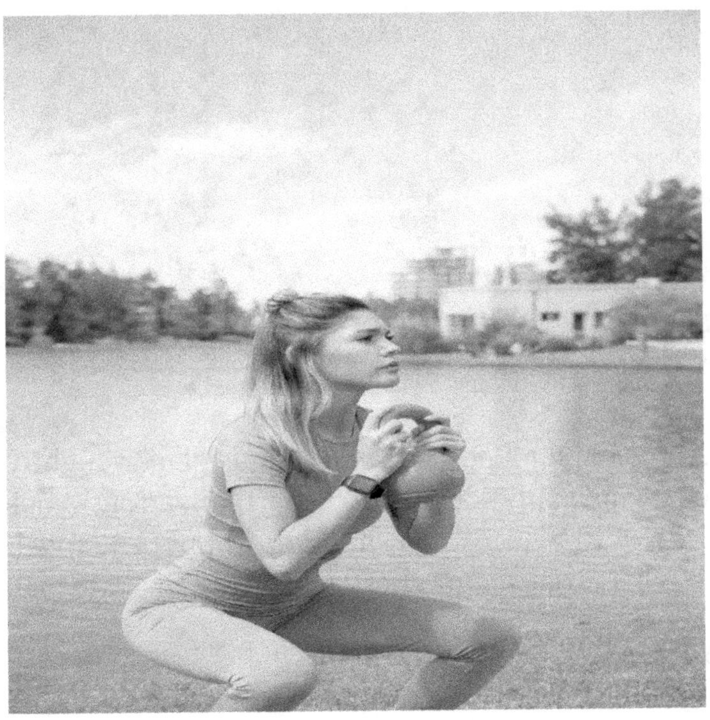

Start with your feet shoulder-width apart, lower your body as if sitting back into an imaginary chair, and then rise back up. This engages your quadriceps, hamstrings, and glutes.

Pro Tip:

Maintain a straight back and avoid letting your knees go past your toes.

2. Push-Ups:

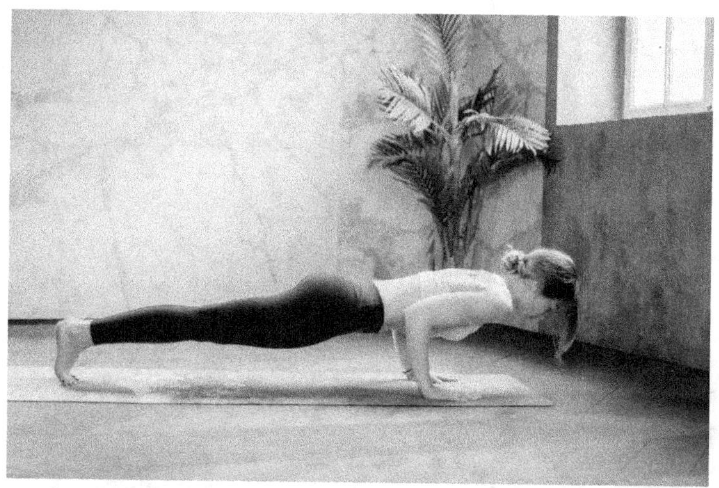

Assume a plank position with hands placed slightly wider than shoulder-width apart. Bending your elbows, lower your body to the ground and push back. This targets your chest, shoulders, and triceps.

Pro Tip:

Keep your body in a straight line from your head to your heels, keeping your core active.

Progression and Consistency

As you embrace strength training, progression is key. Begin with a manageable intensity and gradually increase the challenge. For instance, if you started with ten bodyweight squats, aim for twelve in the following week. Consistency is your ally; make strength training a regular part of your routine to witness sustainable results.

Tailoring Your Routine

Crafting a workout routine tailored to your goals involves understanding muscle groups and selecting exercises that target them effectively. Consider incorporating compound exercises like deadlifts and bench presses to engage multiple muscle groups simultaneously.

Tracking Your Journey

Keeping track of your development is an enlightening and inspiring habit. Whether through a fitness app, journal, or photos, tracking your strength gains provides tangible evidence of your hard work, encouraging you to persevere.

Note.... Building strength is a journey of self-discovery and empowerment. By understanding the fundamentals, maintaining proper form, progressing gradually, and staying consistent, you'll unlock your body's potential for strength and resilience.

3.2: SCULPTING YOUR PHYSIQUE WITH BODY TONING EXERCISE

Welcome to the chapter where we embark on a journey of sculpting, toning, and refining your physique. If you've just joined us from the 30-day Fat Burning Challenge, kudos on completing the first leg of your fitness adventure. Now, let's dive into the realm of body toning exercises – a crucial phase in shaping the physique you desire.

1. Understanding Body Toning

Body toning isn't about bulking up; it's about shaping and defining your muscles while shedding excess fat. It's the art of creating a lean, sculpted physique that mirrors strength and balance. My own transition from fat burning to toning was a natural progression, an evolution in my fitness journey.

2. The Foundation of Body Toning

Before we delve into specific exercises, it's essential to understand the foundation of body toning – building lean muscle. Why does this matter? More muscle mass contributes to a higher resting metabolic rate, meaning you burn more calories even when at rest. It's a win-win – a sculpted body and increased calorie burn.

3. The Role of Nutrition

As we venture into body toning, nutrition plays a pivotal role. It's not about drastic diets but rather fueling your body with the right nutrients. Think of it as providing the necessary building blocks for your muscles. A balanced intake of proteins, carbohydrates, and healthy fats ensures your body has what it needs for muscle development.

Reflecting on my 30-day Challenge, this transition meant tweaking my dietary habits. It wasn't about deprivation but about making choices that fueled my workouts and supported my fitness goals.

4. Body Toning Exercises: The Essentials

Now, let's explore some fundamental body toning exercises. Remember, the aim is to target multiple muscle groups, enhancing overall definition. You don't need fancy equipment – just your determination and perhaps a comfortable workout mat.

Plank Variations: Planks engage the core, arms, and legs. Gradually extend your time and experiment with side planks for added challenge.

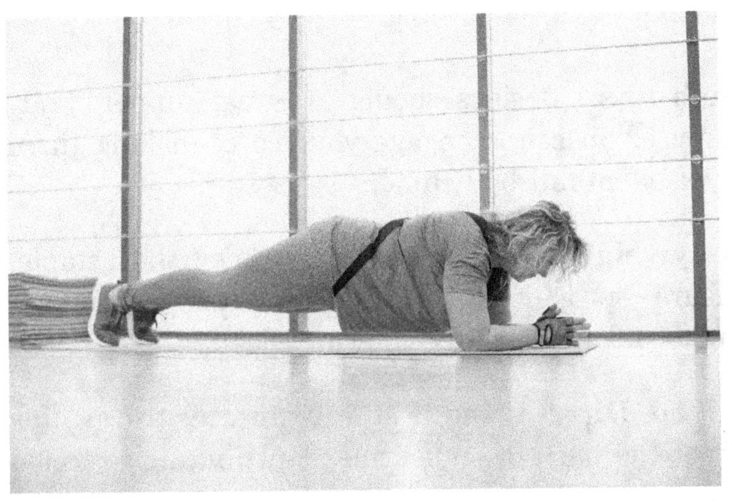

Lunges: Take your lunges up a notch. Forward lunges, reverse lunges, and side lunges all contribute to sculpting your lower body.

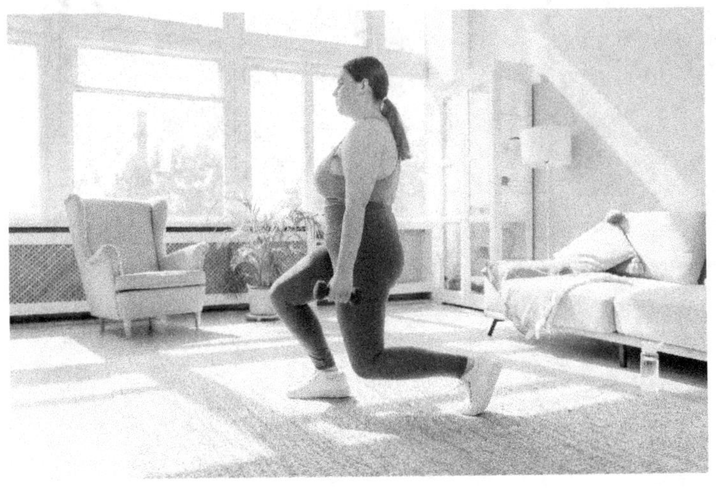

Push-ups: Besides being a great upper body exercise, push-ups engage your core, making them an excellent full-body toner.

Bodyweight Squats: These continue to be a staple. Ensure proper form and gradually increase repetitions to challenge your muscles.

Tricep Dips: Using a sturdy surface, tricep dips target the back of your arms, contributing to toned arms.

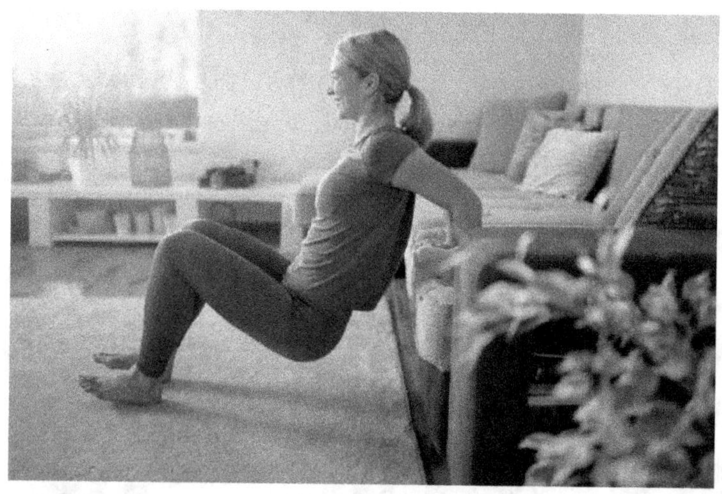

5. The Art of Reps and Sets

Effective toning requires a strategic approach to repetitions (reps) and sets. Aim for moderate reps with a focus on proper form. For beginners, starting with 2-3 sets of 10-15 reps per exercise is a good foundation. As you progress, you can adjust based on your comfort and fitness level.

6. Progression in Toning

Just as with the Fat Burning Challenge, progression is key in body toning. Gradually increase the intensity of your exercises – more reps, challenging variations, or incorporating light weights if you feel ready. This progression prevents plateaus and keeps your muscles adapting.

7. Consistency is key

Consistency remains the backbone of any fitness journey. Body toning is a gradual process, and the magic happens when you consistently incorporate these exercises into your routine. My journey taught me that visible changes take time, but the commitment pays off.

8. Embracing the Sculpted Lifestyle

Body toning isn't a temporary fix; it's a lifestyle. It's about finding joy in movement, embracing strength, and appreciating the capability of your body. As you sculpt your physique, relish in the process and acknowledge the progress along the way.

9. Listen to Your Body

Throughout this chapter and your fitness journey, remember to listen to your body. If an exercise doesn't feel right or if you need an extra day of rest, that's perfectly okay. Fitness is about nurturing your body, not pushing it to the brink.

10. Celebrate Milestones

Whether it's holding a plank for an extra 10 seconds or noticing increased definition in your arms, celebrate these milestones. They signify your dedication and the positive changes happening within.

11. Closing Thoughts

As we wrap up this chapter on body toning, envision the sculpted physique you're working towards. It's not about conforming to societal standards but about feeling strong, confident, and healthy in your own skin. This journey is yours – sculpt it with intention, embrace the process, and let's continue shaping a healthier, toned you. The adventure continues.

3.3: CARDIOVASCULAR FITNESS FOR BEGINNERS

In the journey towards a healthier lifestyle, cardiovascular fitness plays a pivotal role in enhancing overall well-being. This chapter explores the fundamentals of cardiovascular fitness for beginners, drawing inspiration from a 30-day Fat Burning Challenge tailored for total beginners, all without the need for specialized exercise equipment.

The Basics of Cardiovascular Fitness

Before delving into the specifics of the 30-day challenge, let's establish a solid understanding of cardiovascular fitness. At its core, cardiovascular fitness refers to the efficiency with which our heart, lungs, and blood vessels work together to supply oxygen and nutrients to the body during physical activity.

Key Components:

1. Heart Health: The heart, our body's engine, pumps blood efficiently, ensuring oxygen is delivered to muscles.

2. Lung Capacity: Improved lung function enhances the intake of oxygen, vital for sustained physical activity.

3. Circulation: Efficient blood flow ensures nutrients reach muscles and waste products are removed.

My Personal Journey: The 30-Day Fat Burning Challenge

Embarking on a 30-day Fat Burning Challenge for total beginners was a transformative experience. This challenge focused on accessible exercises, making it ideal for those new to fitness. The absence of equipment eliminated barriers, allowing anyone to participate and reap the benefits of cardiovascular exercise.

Day 1-5: Establishing a Routine

The initial days centered around creating a consistent workout routine. Simple exercises like brisk walking, jumping jacks, and stair climbing were incorporated, laying the foundation for increased heart rate and improved circulation. Each day built upon the previous, gradually elevating the intensity.

Day 6-15: Introducing High-Intensity Interval Training (HIIT)

As the body adapted, the challenge integrated High-Intensity Interval Training (HIIT). Short bursts of intense activity alternated with brief periods of rest, boosting metabolism and enhancing cardiovascular endurance. Exercises like burpees, mountain climbers, and high knees added variety and intensity to the routine.

Day 16-30: Building Endurance

The latter part of the challenge focused on building endurance. Longer sessions of brisk walking or jogging, combined with bodyweight exercises, pushed boundaries and enhanced cardiovascular stamina. Progress became evident not only in physical endurance but also in increased energy levels and a sense of accomplishment.

The Importance of Clear Communication

Communicating the benefits of cardiovascular fitness is crucial, especially for beginners. Clear language and descriptive examples make the journey more comprehensible. Consider the following:

1. **Metabolic Boost**: Cardiovascular exercise increases metabolism, aiding in weight management. Imagine your body as a well-tuned

engine burning calories efficiently during and after workouts.

2. Stress Reduction: Regular cardiovascular activity releases endorphins, reducing stress and enhancing mental well-being. Picture the calming effect of a post-workout walk or jog.

3. Heart Health: Improved circulation lowers the risk of heart disease. Visualize your heart pumping efficiently, ensuring optimal health and longevity.

Incorporating Variety for Motivation

To keep the journey engaging, incorporate a variety of activities. Consider cycling, swimming, or dance workouts. Diversity not only prevents monotony but also targets different muscle groups, promoting overall fitness.

Cardiovascular fitness for beginners is not just a physical endeavor but a holistic approach to well-being. My 30-day Fat Burning Challenge exemplifies that with commitment, consistency, and clear communication, anyone can embark on a transformative fitness journey. Remember, it's not just about the destination; it's about enjoying the journey towards a healthier, more vibrant you.

3.4: FLEXIBILITY and MOBILITY ESSENTIALS

In the pursuit of overall fitness, flexibility and mobility are often overlooked but are essential components that contribute to a well-rounded and functional body. This chapter delves into the fundamentals of flexibility and mobility, drawing inspiration from my personal experience in a 30-day Fat Burning Challenge for total beginners, emphasizing the importance of these aspects alongside cardiovascular fitness.

Understanding Flexibility and Mobility

Before we explore the specifics, let's grasp the concepts of flexibility and mobility.

Flexibility:

The range of motion around a joint is referred to as flexibility. It involves the ability of muscles and connective tissues to stretch, allowing joints to move through their full range.

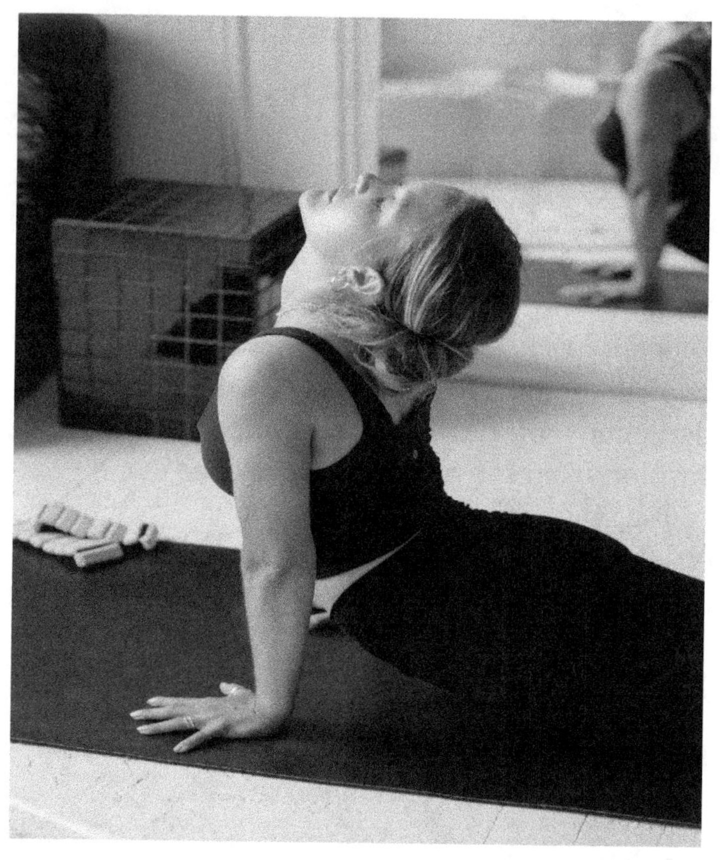

Mobility:

Mobility is the functional capacity of joints to move freely through their intended range. It encompasses flexibility but goes beyond, emphasizing control and stability during movement.

My Personal Journey: A Holistic Approach

While navigating the 30-day Fat Burning Challenge, I quickly realized the significance of flexibility and mobility. The initial focus on cardiovascular exercises set the stage, but it became evident that a holistic approach to fitness included the ability to move freely and efficiently.

Day 1-10: Foundation of Flexibility

The first ten days introduced basic flexibility exercises to the routine. Simple stretches like toe touches, seated hamstring stretches, and shoulder rotations helped increase flexibility gradually. The aim was not only to improve the range of motion but also to reduce the risk of injury during more dynamic exercises.

Day 11-20: Enhancing Mobility

As the challenge progressed, emphasis shifted to mobility exercises. Dynamic movements such as leg swings, arm circles, and hip rotations were introduced. These exercises not only enhanced joint mobility but also improved coordination, contributing to a more fluid and controlled movement pattern.

Day 21-30: Fusion of Flexibility and Mobility

In the final phase, a fusion of flexibility and mobility exercises was incorporated. Yoga-inspired flows and Pilates movements seamlessly integrated stretches with dynamic actions. This combination not only promoted a balanced range of motion but also improved overall body awareness and control.

The Significance of Flexibility

Understanding the importance of flexibility is pivotal for any fitness journey. Consider the following key points:

1. Injury Prevention: Improved flexibility reduces the likelihood of injuries by allowing the body to move more naturally and efficiently.

2. Posture Improvement: Flexibility contributes to better posture, aligning the body correctly and reducing strain on muscles and joints.

3. Enhanced Performance: Whether in daily activities or during workouts, increased flexibility enhances overall performance by optimizing movement patterns.

Mobility's Role in Functional Fitness

Mobility is the unsung hero of functional fitness. It goes beyond static stretches and addresses the body's ability to move with purpose. Here's why mobility matters:

1. Joint Health: Regular mobility exercises promote optimal joint health by lubricating joints and preventing stiffness.

2. Improved Balance and Coordination: Enhanced mobility contributes to better balance and coordination, crucial for daily activities and preventing falls.

3. Functional Movement: Mobility exercises replicate real-life movements, ensuring your body is well-equipped for the demands of everyday life.

Incorporating Flexibility and Mobility into Your Routine

Now that we understand the importance of flexibility and mobility, let's explore practical ways to incorporate these into our fitness routine:

1. Warm-Up with Dynamic Stretches: Start your workouts with dynamic stretches to prepare your muscles and joints for activity.

2. Dedicate Time to Stretching: Allocate specific time for static stretching, focusing on major muscle groups after your workout.

3. Include Mobility Drills: Integrate dynamic movements into your routine, incorporating exercises that mimic daily activities.

Conclusion

Incorporating flexibility and mobility into your fitness journey is not an option; it's a necessity. My experience in the 30-day Fat Burning Challenge illuminated the symbiotic relationship between cardiovascular fitness, flexibility, and mobility. By embracing a comprehensive approach, you not only enhance your physical capabilities but also promote long-term health and well-being. As we move forward in our fitness endeavors, let's remember that a body in motion, with flexibility and mobility at its core, is a body that thrives.

3.5: INCORPORATING FUNCTIONAL TRAINING

Functional training, often hailed as the bridge between exercise and real-life movements, is a key element in building a resilient and adaptable body. In this chapter, we'll explore the fundamentals of functional training, drawing insights from my personal experience in the 30-day Fat Burning Challenge for total beginners. This regimen not only focused on cardiovascular fitness, flexibility, and mobility but also highlighted the importance of functional training for a well-rounded and practical approach to exercise.

Understanding Functional Training

Functional training revolves around exercises that mimic everyday movements and activities, emphasizing the integration of various muscle groups and promoting overall body functionality. Unlike isolated exercises, functional training enhances the body's ability to perform tasks efficiently in real-life scenarios.

My Personal Journey: The Evolution of Fitness

As the 30-day Fat Burning Challenge progressed, I discovered that functional training was the missing link for a comprehensive fitness routine. Here's how it seamlessly integrated into the challenge:

Day 1-10: Foundation Building

The initial phase of the challenge established a foundation for functional movements. Bodyweight exercises like squats, lunges, and push-ups became staples, promoting strength and stability in a way that echoed natural motions.

Day 11-20: Dynamic Integration

As the challenge advanced, dynamic movements were introduced. Exercises such as bear crawls, plank variations, and rotational lunges not only elevated the heart rate but also engaged multiple muscle groups simultaneously, mimicking the complexity of daily movements.

Day 21-30: Everyday Functionality

In the final stretch, the challenge incorporated exercises inspired by daily activities. Functional movements like carrying groceries, mimicking picking up a child, and performing agility drills were integrated. This not only added variety but also demonstrated the practical application of functional training.

The Key Principles of Functional Training

To grasp the essence of functional training, let's explore its core principles:

1. Multi-Planar Movements:

Functional exercises occur in multiple planes of motion, replicating the diverse ways our bodies move in daily life. This includes forward and backward, side-to-side, and rotational movements.

2.Engaging Core Stability:

Functional training places a strong emphasis on core stability. A stable core is the foundation for most movements, contributing to overall strength and balance.

3. Integration of Multiple Muscle Groups:

Unlike isolation exercises that target specific muscles, functional training involves the coordination of various muscle groups. This mirrors the synergistic nature of our body's movements.

The Practical Benefits of Functional Training

Now that we understand the principles, let's explore the tangible benefits of incorporating functional training into your fitness routine:

1. Improved Daily Functionality:

Functional training enhances your ability to perform daily tasks with ease, from lifting groceries to bending down to tie your shoelaces.

2. Enhanced Stability and Balance:

Engaging multiple muscle groups in a coordinated manner improves overall stability and balance, reducing the risk of falls and injuries.

3. Efficient Caloric Burn:

Functional exercises often involve full-body movements, resulting in a higher caloric burn compared to isolated exercises, contributing to weight management.

Incorporating Functional Training Into Your Routine

Making functional training a part of your regular exercise routine doesn't have to be complicated. Here are practical ways to incorporate it:

1. Bodyweight Exercises:

Start with foundational bodyweight exercises like squats, lunges, and push-ups, ensuring proper form and gradually increasing intensity.

2. Functional Movements:

Include dynamic movements such as bear crawls, planks with shoulder taps, and mountain climbers to engage various muscle groups simultaneously.

3. Daily Activity Integration:

Identify opportunities to incorporate functional movements inspired by daily activities. For example, practice squatting while picking up objects from the ground or performing lunges while carrying a backpack.

Realizing the Synergy

As I navigated the 30-day Fat Burning Challenge, the synergy between functional training, cardiovascular fitness, flexibility, and mobility became apparent. Here's how functional training complements the other aspects:

1. Functional Cardiovascular Training:

Dynamic movements in functional training elevate the heart rate, providing a cardiovascular workout that is both efficient and practical.

2. Flexibility and Mobility Integration:

Functional training promotes flexibility and mobility by engaging muscles and joints in a variety of movements, enhancing range of motion and reducing stiffness.

Embracing a Holistic Fitness Approach

In conclusion, incorporating functional training into your fitness routine is not just about building strength; it's about preparing your body for the demands of everyday life. My journey in the 30-day Fat Burning Challenge emphasized that true fitness is a synergy of various elements. By embracing functional training, you not only enhance your physical capabilities but also cultivate a body that is resilient, adaptable, and ready for whatever life throws at it. As you continue on your fitness journey, remember that each movement is a step towards a stronger, more functional you.

CHAPTER 4
4.1: DESIGNING EFFECTIVE WORKOUT SPLITS

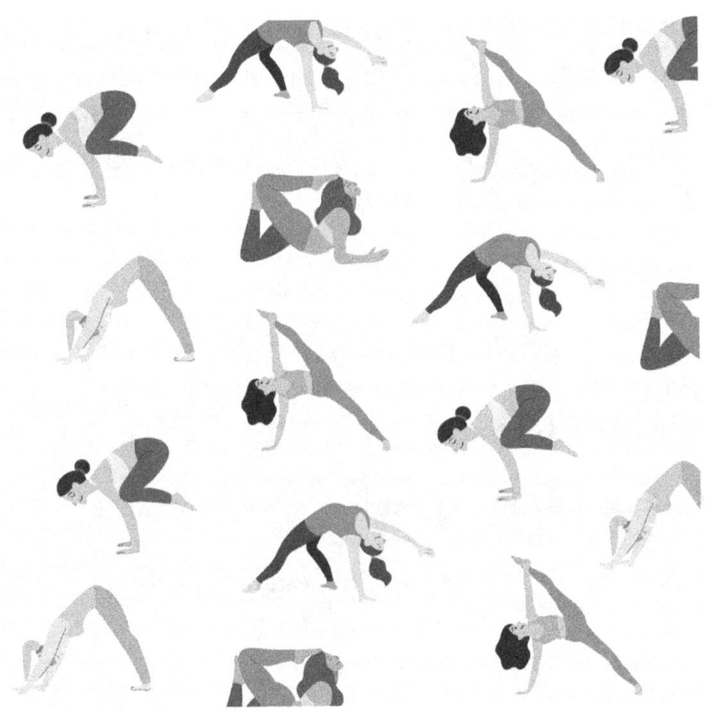

Embarking on a fitness journey requires more than just enthusiasm; it demands a well-structured plan. This chapter explores the intricacies of designing effective workout splits, drawing insights from my personal experience in the 30-day Fat Burning

Challenge for total beginners. Understanding how to organize your workouts optimally can significantly contribute to achieving your fitness goals.

The Importance of Workout Splits

Before diving into the nitty-gritty of workout splits, let's understand why they matter. A workout split refers to the way you organize and distribute your exercises throughout the week. Properly designed splits offer several advantages:

1. Muscle Recovery:

Allowing specific muscle groups to rest while working others prevents overtraining and promotes effective recovery.

2. Consistent Progress:

Structured splits ensure that each muscle group is targeted with sufficient intensity and frequency, promoting consistent progress.

3. Adaptability:

Tailoring your workout splits to your goals—whether it's strength, endurance, or overall fitness—provides a roadmap for your fitness journey.

My Personal Journey: The Evolution of Workout Splits

In the initial phase of the 30-day Fat Burning Challenge, the focus was on full-body workouts to introduce beginners to various exercises. As the challenge progressed, a more detailed approach to workout splits emerged:

Day 1-10: Full-Body Foundation

The initial days of the challenge incorporated full-body workouts. Exercises like bodyweight squats, push-ups, and planks engaged multiple muscle groups, providing a foundational understanding of different movements.

Day 11-20: Upper/Lower Split

As participants gained familiarity with exercises, the challenge transitioned into an upper/lower split. Days dedicated to upper body exercises alternated with days focusing on lower body exercises. This allowed specific muscle groups to recover while others were engaged.

Day 21-30: Targeted Muscle Group Splits

In the final phase, the challenge adopted a targeted approach. Specific days were allocated to different muscle groups—for instance, chest and triceps, back and biceps, legs, and core. This refined split targeted muscles more precisely, promoting both strength and endurance.

Designing Your Workout Splits

Now, let's explore the steps to design effective workout splits tailored to your fitness goals:

1. Determine Your Goals:

Identify your fitness objectives—whether it's building muscle, improving endurance, or achieving overall fitness. Your goals will shape the structure of your workout splits.

2. Consider Your Schedule:

Take into account how many days a week you can dedicate to exercise. Your split should align with your availability to ensure consistency.

3. Understand Different Splits:

Explore various workout splits such as full-body, upper/lower, push/pull, or specific muscle group splits. Each has its advantages, and the choice depends on your goals and preferences.

4. Include Rest Days:

Rest is a crucial component of any workout split. Adequate rest days allow your muscles to recover, preventing burnout and reducing the risk of injuries.

Tailoring Splits to Your Goals

Let's break down how different workout splits align with specific fitness goals:

1. Full-Body Splits:

Ideal for beginners and those aiming for overall fitness. Each session engages multiple muscle groups, promoting a balanced approach.

2. Upper/Lower Splits:

Suited for those looking to build strength and increase muscle mass. This split allows focused training on upper and lower body muscles, promoting recovery.

3. Push/Pull Splits:

Effective for individuals targeting specific muscle groups, such as chest and triceps (push) or back and biceps (pull). This split offers targeted training for muscle definition.

4. Specific Muscle Group Splits:

Perfect for advanced fitness enthusiasts aiming to focus on individual muscle groups. This split allows for detailed training, emphasizing specific areas of the body.

Sample Weekly Workout Split

Let's put theory into practice with a sample workout split:

Day 1: Full-Body Workout

- Squats

- Push-ups

- Plank

- Lunges

Day 2: Rest

Day 3: Upper/Lower Split

- Upper Body: Bench Press, Rows, Bicep Curls

- Lower Body: Deadlifts, Leg Press, Calf Raises

Day 4: Rest or Light Activity

Day 5: Push/Pull Split

- Push: Shoulder Press, Tricep Dips

- Pull: Pull-Ups, Bent-Over Rows

Day 6: Rest or Light Activity

Day 7: Specific Muscle Group Split

- Chest and Triceps: Chest Flyes, Tricep Kickbacks

- Back and Biceps: Lat Pulldowns, Bicep Hammer Curls

The Importance of Adaptation

As your fitness journey progresses, be open to adapting your workout splits. Listen to your body and adjust based on your evolving goals, preferences, and lifestyle changes. Flexibility in your routine ensures sustained motivation and prevents plateaus.

Conclusion

Designing effective workout splits is akin to crafting a roadmap for your fitness journey. My experience in the 30-day Fat Burning Challenge highlighted that a well-thought-out split not only enhances the effectiveness of your workouts but also contributes to long-term progress. As you embark on your fitness endeavors, remember that the key lies in aligning your splits with your goals, maintaining consistency, and embracing the adaptability needed for a sustainable and successful fitness journey.

4.2 : PROGRESSION TECHNIQUES FOR CONTINUOUS IMPROVEMENTS

Embarking on a fitness journey is not just about starting; it's about evolving and progressing. In this chapter, we'll delve into essential progression techniques, drawing insights from my personal experience in the 30-day Fat Burning Challenge for total beginners. Understanding how to continually challenge your body is the key to sustained improvement and long-term success in your fitness endeavors.

The Significance of Progression

Progression is the heartbeat of fitness. It goes beyond simply going through the motions; it involves pushing boundaries and challenging your body to adapt. Here's why progression matters:

1. Avoiding Plateaus:

Progression prevents plateaus by introducing new challenges, ensuring your body doesn't become accustomed to a routine.

2. Building Strength and Endurance:

Gradual progression builds strength and endurance over time, allowing you to take on more challenging exercises and activities.

3. Sustaining Motivation:

Achieving new milestones keeps motivation alive. Progression transforms your fitness journey into a dynamic and rewarding experience.

My Personal Journey: Unveiling the Power of Progression

The 30-day Fat Burning Challenge was a testament to the transformative power of progression. Here's how the challenge evolved, incorporating various techniques to keep the momentum going:

Day 1-10: Establishing Baseline Fitness

The initial phase focused on establishing a baseline fitness level. Basic exercises were introduced, allowing beginners to get comfortable with movements. The aim was to create a foundation for progression.

Day 11-20: Increasing Intensity

As participants adapted to the workouts, intensity levels were gradually increased. For example, bodyweight squats progressed to jump squats, and regular planks evolved into plank variations. Incremental changes elevated the challenge without overwhelming participants.

Day 21-30: Introducing Time and Repetition Challenges

In the final stretch, the challenge incorporated time and repetition challenges. For instance, participants were encouraged to complete more rounds of exercises within a set time or increase the number of repetitions. This not only added a competitive edge but also pushed individuals to surpass their previous limits.

Techniques for Effective Progression

Let's explore specific techniques to incorporate into your fitness routine for continuous improvement:

1. Incremental Load Increases:

Increase the weight or resistance in your workouts gradually. This can be achieved by adding a few extra pounds, incorporating resistance bands, or progressing to more advanced variations.

2. Time Under Tension:

Control the pace of your exercises, emphasizing the time your muscles spend under tension. Slowing down movements increases the intensity, fostering muscle engagement and growth.

3. Progressive Overload:

Systematically increase the difficulty of your workouts. This can be achieved by adding more sets, repetitions, or incorporating more challenging exercises.

4. Variation and Complexity:

Introduce variety into your routine. Experiment with different exercises and their variations to challenge your muscles in new ways. Complex movements engage multiple muscle groups, promoting overall development.

5. Rest-Pause Technique:

During your workout, take short breaks between sets to extend the overall duration of your exercise session. This technique increases the intensity of your workout without compromising form.

6. Periodization:

Organize your training into different phases with varying intensities. For example, have periods of high-intensity workouts followed by phases of active recovery. This helps prevent burnout and promotes long-term progression.

Sample Progression Plan

Let's create a sample progression plan for a basic bodyweight exercise:

Exercise: Bodyweight Squats

1. Baseline (Day 1-10):

Perform 3 sets of 12 squats.

2. Increased Intensity (Day 11-20):

Increase sets to 4 and repetitions to 15.

3. Time and Repetition Challenge (Day 21-30):

Complete as many squats as possible in one minute or aim for 5 sets of 20 squats.

Avoiding Common Pitfalls

While progression is essential, it's crucial to avoid common pitfalls that could hinder your journey. Here are a few things to watch out for:

1. Too Rapid Progression:

Gradual progression is key. Jumping to advanced exercises or significantly increasing intensity too quickly can lead to injuries.

2. Ignoring Recovery:

Progression is not only about pushing harder; it's also about allowing your body to recover. Neglecting rest can lead to burnout and hinder progress.

3. Neglecting Form:

Maintain proper form, especially when introducing new exercises or increasing intensity. Sacrificing form for the sake of progression increases the risk of injuries.

Celebrating Milestones

As you implement progression techniques, celebrate the milestones along the way. Whether it's completing an extra set, achieving a personal best in repetitions, or mastering a challenging exercise, acknowledging your progress reinforces your commitment and motivates you to reach new heights.

Conclusion

Progression is the heartbeat of a successful fitness journey. My experience in the 30-day Fat Burning Challenge highlighted that continuous improvement is not just about working harder; it's about working smarter. By incorporating thoughtful progression techniques, you not only challenge your body but also cultivate a mindset of growth and resilience. As you navigate your fitness journey, remember that each step forward, no matter how small, brings you closer to the healthier and stronger version of yourself. Embrace progression, celebrate your victories, and let the journey unfold one positive change at a time.

4.3 : BALANCING CARDIO and STRENGTH TRAINING

Achieving a harmonious balance between cardiovascular (cardio) exercise and strength training is at the core of a well-rounded fitness routine. In this chapter, we'll explore the importance of striking this balance, drawing insights from my personal experience in the 30-day Fat Burning Challenge for total beginners. Understanding how to integrate cardio and strength training not only enhances your overall fitness but also contributes to a healthier and more resilient body.

The Symbiotic Relationship

Cardiovascular exercise and strength training, often seen as distinct components of fitness, share a symbiotic relationship. Balancing these two elements is crucial for comprehensive well-being. Let's delve into why this synergy matters:

1. Cardiovascular Health:

Cardio exercises like running, cycling, or brisk walking elevate your heart rate, improving circulation and cardiovascular health.

2. Strength and Muscle Development:

Strength training, on the other hand, focuses on building muscle, enhancing bone density, and boosting metabolism.

My Personal Journey: Navigating the Balance

The 30-day Fat Burning Challenge showcased the interplay between cardio and strength training. Here's how the challenge integrated both components:

Day 1-10: Cardio Foundation

The initial phase incorporated cardio exercises to establish a foundation. Activities like jumping jacks, high knees, and jogging in place elevated the heart rate, preparing the body for more intense workouts.

Day 11-20: Introduction of Strength Training

As participants adapted, strength training exercises were gradually introduced. Bodyweight exercises like squats, lunges, and push-ups targeted different muscle groups, complementing the cardiovascular workouts.

Day 21-30: Fusion of Cardio and Strength

In the final phase, the challenge seamlessly blended cardio and strength exercises. High-Intensity Interval Training (HIIT) sessions became a staple, combining bursts of intense cardio with bodyweight strength exercises for a holistic workout.

The Benefits of Cardiovascular Exercise

Let's explore the specific advantages of incorporating cardiovascular exercise into your routine:

1. Improved Heart Health:

Cardio activities strengthen the heart, enhancing its ability to pump blood efficiently and reducing the risk of heart disease.

2. Caloric Burn and Weight Management:

Cardio exercises contribute to calorie burning, aiding in weight management and fat loss when combined with a balanced diet.

3. Increased Stamina:

Regular cardio workouts improve endurance, allowing you to engage in physical activities for more extended periods without fatigue.

The Benefits of Strength Training

Similarly, strength training offers a multitude of benefits that enhance overall fitness:

1. Muscle and Bone Health:

Strength training stimulates muscle growth, improves muscle tone, and enhances bone density, promoting long-term skeletal health.

2. Metabolism Boost:

Building lean muscle mass boosts metabolism, helping your body burn more calories even at rest.

3. Injury Prevention:

Strength training improves joint stability and flexibility, reducing the risk of injuries during physical activities.

Crafting a Balanced Routine

Now, let's explore how to create a balanced routine that incorporates both cardio and strength training:

1. Establish Clear Goals:

Define your fitness goals, whether they are weight loss, muscle building, or overall well-being. Your goals will guide the intensity and frequency of your workouts.

2. Mix Up Your Cardio Workouts:

Incorporate a variety of cardio exercises to keep your routine engaging. This could include running, cycling, swimming, or even dance workouts.

3. Integrate Strength Training:

Include strength training exercises at least two to three times a week. Focus on major muscle groups, including legs, back, chest, arms, and core.

4. HIIT Workouts for Efficiency:

High-Intensity Interval Training (HIIT) is an efficient way to blend cardio and strength. Short bursts of intense activity followed by brief rests provide both cardiovascular benefits and strength building.

Sample Weekly Routine

Let's create a sample weekly routine that balances cardio and strength training:

Monday:

- Cardio: 30 minutes of brisk walking or jogging

- Strength: Bodyweight squats, push-ups, and planks (3 sets of 12-15 repetitions)

Wednesday:

- Cardio: Cycling or swimming for 30 minutes

- Strength: Lunges, tricep dips, and mountain climbers (3 sets of 12-15 repetitions)

Friday:

- HIIT Workout:

- Jumping jacks, burpees, and high knees (30 seconds each, repeated for 3 rounds)

- Strength: Deadlifts, bicep curls, and Russian twists (3 sets of 12-15 repetitions)

Listen to Your Body

While a balanced routine is essential, it's equally crucial to listen to your body. Pay attention to signs of fatigue or discomfort and modify your workouts accordingly. Adequate rest and recovery are integral to sustained progress.

Celebrating Milestones in Balance

As you balance cardio and strength training, celebrate the milestones achieved in both realms. Whether it's completing a longer run, lifting heavier weights, or achieving a personal best in a cardio-strength fusion workout, each achievement is a step towards a healthier you.

Conclusion

Balancing cardio and strength training is not about choosing one over the other; it's about recognizing the symbiotic relationship between the two and crafting a routine that optimally blends both elements. My journey in the 30-day Fat Burning Challenge underscored the transformative power of this balance. As you navigate your fitness journey, remember that a well-rounded approach contributes to overall health, resilience, and a sense of accomplishment. Embrace the synergy between cardio and strength training, celebrate your progress, and revel in the vitality of a body that thrives on a harmonious blend of movement and strength.

4.4: REST and RECOVERY - A Vital Component

In the journey toward a healthier lifestyle, rest and recovery often take a backseat to the more energetic aspects of fitness. However, their significance cannot be overstated. This chapter explores the crucial role that rest and recovery play in achieving sustainable fitness goals, drawing insights from my own 30-day Fat Burning Challenge tailored for total beginners without the need for exercise equipment.

Understanding the Importance of Rest

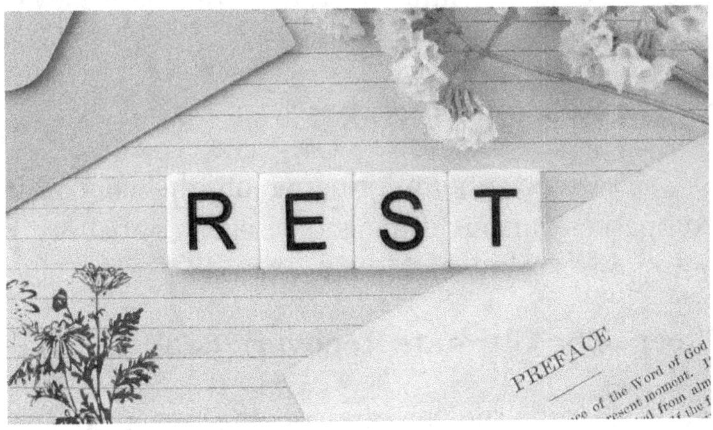

Before delving into the specifics of recovery, it's essential to grasp why adequate rest is integral to any fitness regimen. Imagine your body as a well-oiled machine; it needs downtime to repair, rebuild, and recalibrate. Without sufficient rest, the risk of burnout and injuries escalates, undermining your progress.

Personal Experience: The Turning Point

During my 30-day Fat Burning Challenge, I initially underestimated the importance of rest days. Pushing through consecutive workouts led to fatigue, affecting both my physical and mental well-being. Recognizing this, I adjusted my approach, incorporating rest days strategically. The impact on my energy levels and overall performance was remarkable.

Types of Rest and Recovery

Rest isn't solely about lounging on the couch; it encompasses various dimensions, each contributing to your body's rejuvenation.

1. Sleep: The Ultimate Recovery Tool

Quality sleep is the linchpin of effective recovery. During the 30-day challenge, I realized the transformative power of a good night's sleep. It aids muscle repair, regulates hormones, and enhances cognitive function. Consider it your secret weapon for optimal performance.

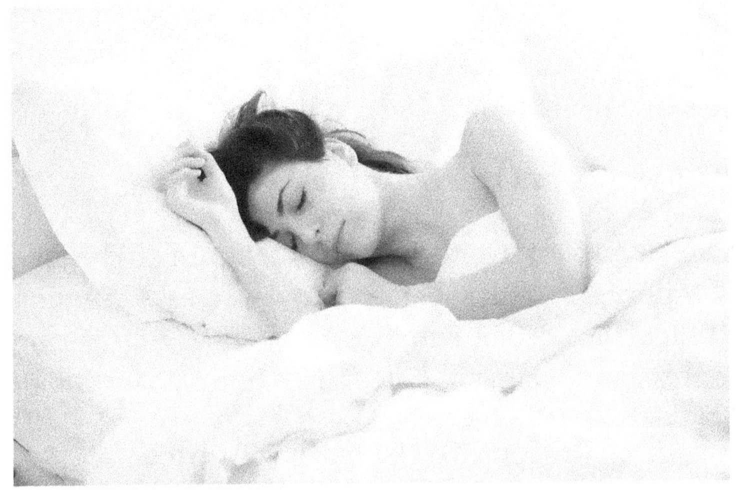

2. Active Recovery: Gentle Movement Matters

Contrary to popular belief, recovery doesn't always mean complete inactivity. Incorporating light activities like walking or yoga on rest days promotes blood circulation, reduces muscle stiffness, and fosters a sense of well-being.

3. Nutrition: Fueling Your Recovery

An essential part of the healing process is nutrition. Reflecting on my challenge, I discovered the significance of post-workout nutrition. Incorporating protein-rich snacks facilitated muscle recovery and replenished energy stores, ensuring I was ready for the next session.

The Pitfalls of Overtraining

In the pursuit of fitness goals, it's tempting to believe that more is always better. However, overtraining can lead to detrimental consequences, hindering progress and increasing the risk of injury.

Personal Reflection: Finding Balance

Through my 30-day challenge, I learned the art of balance. Pushing myself without heed resulted in setbacks. Embracing a balanced approach that includes rest and recovery allowed me to achieve sustainable results, setting the foundation for long-term success.

Crafting Your Rest and Recovery Plan

Armed with the knowledge of the importance of rest and recovery, it's time to personalize your approach. Consider the following steps to optimize your recovery:

1. Listen to Your Body:

Pay attention to signals of fatigue, soreness, and stress. Adjust your workout intensity and schedule accordingly.

2. Schedule Rest Days:

Plan regular rest days into your routine. Treat them with the same importance as your workout sessions.

3. Hydrate and Nourish:

Adequate hydration and proper nutrition are crucial components of recovery. Make sure you are providing the nutrition your body requires. Prioritize Sleep:

Establish a consistent sleep schedule. Quality sleep is essential for effective recovery.

4.5: ADAPTING THE PROGRAM FOR LONG-TERM SUCCESS

Embarking on a fitness program is not just a short-term commitment; it's a journey toward lasting well-being. In this chapter, we'll explore the importance of adapting your fitness program for long-term success, drawing insights from my personal experience in the 30-day Fat Burning Challenge for total beginners. Understanding how to make sustainable adjustments ensures that your fitness journey remains dynamic and enjoyable as you progress toward your health and fitness goals.

The Evolution of a Fitness Program

A successful fitness program is not static; it evolves with your changing needs, goals, and lifestyle. Adapting your program ensures continued motivation, prevents plateaus, and accommodates the dynamic nature of life. Here's how you can approach this evolution:

Reflecting on Your Goals

Begin by revisiting your initial fitness goals. Whether it's weight loss, muscle building, or improved overall health, understanding your objectives is crucial for making informed adjustments. Your goals act as the compass guiding your fitness journey.

My Personal Journey: A Dynamic Challenge

The 30-day Fat Burning Challenge exemplified the need for adaptability. As the challenge progressed, it became evident that participants needed modifications based on individual fitness levels, preferences, and goals.

Individualized Adjustments

Participants with different fitness backgrounds adapted the challenge to suit their needs. Some increased the intensity for faster results, while others focused on gradual progress to accommodate physical limitations.

Exploration of Preferences

The challenge incorporated a variety of exercises to cater to different preferences. For instance, those who enjoyed outdoor activities embraced running or cycling, while others preferred indoor exercises like dance workouts.

Goal Reassessment

As participants experienced initial successes, they often reassessed their goals. Some shifted from weight loss to muscle building, while others aimed to enhance overall endurance. This flexibility allowed for continuous engagement.

Key Principles for Long-Term Adaptation

Now, let's explore key principles for adapting your fitness program for long-term success:

1. Gradual Progression:

Avoid sudden, drastic changes. Gradual progression allows your body to adapt, reducing the risk of injuries and ensuring sustainable improvements.

2. Individualization:

Recognize that one size does not fit all. Adapt your program to your individual preferences, fitness level, and any existing health conditions.

3. Consistency Over Perfection:

Consistency trumps perfection. Rather than aiming for flawless adherence, focus on maintaining a consistent routine that aligns with your lifestyle.

4. Periodic Evaluations:

Regularly evaluate your progress and reassess your goals. This allows you to make informed adjustments based on your achievements and evolving priorities.

5. Enjoyable Activities:

Choose activities you genuinely enjoy. If you look forward to your workouts, you're more likely to stay committed in the long run.

Tailoring Cardiovascular Fitness

Adaptation 1:

Exploring Various Cardio Activities

If your initial cardio routine involves running but you find it monotonous, consider exploring alternative activities. Try cycling, swimming, or dance workouts to keep things exciting.

Adaptation 2:

Adjusting Intensity

For sustained cardiovascular benefits, gradually increase the intensity of your workouts. This could involve adding intervals, incorporating hills during a run, or increasing resistance in cycling.

Enhancing Strength Training

Adaptation 1:

Progressing in Weight

As your strength improves, gradually increase the resistance in your strength training exercises. This could mean using heavier weights or exploring advanced bodyweight variations.

Adaptation 2:

Varying Exercises

Prevent boredom and target different muscle groups by introducing new strength training exercises. Experiment with variations to keep your routine engaging and challenging.

Flexibility and Mobility Adjustments

Adaptation 1:

Incorporating Yoga or Pilates

To enhance flexibility and mobility, consider incorporating yoga or Pilates into your routine. These practices not only improve range of motion but also contribute to mental well-being.

Adaptation 2:

Adding Mobility Drills

Integrate specific mobility drills to address areas of stiffness or tightness. Focus on movements that mimic daily activities to enhance overall functional flexibility.

Balancing Cardio and Strength Training

Adaptation 1:

Modifying Intensity and Frequency

Adjust the intensity and frequency of your cardio and strength workouts based on your evolving goals. For instance, you might increase strength training frequency during a muscle-building phase.

Adaptation 2: Experimenting with Combined Workouts

Explore workouts that seamlessly blend cardio and strength training, such as circuit training or CrossFit-style routines. This approach not only saves time but also provides a well-rounded fitness experience.

Sustainable Progression

Adapting to Time Constraints

Adaptation 1:

Shorter, Intense Workouts

If time constraints arise, opt for shorter but more intense workouts. High-Intensity Interval Training (HIIT) is an excellent choice, offering cardiovascular and strength benefits in a condensed timeframe.

Adaptation 2:

Splitting Workouts

Consider splitting your workouts throughout the day. A morning cardio session and an evening strength workout can be just as effective and more manageable.

Adapting to Life Changes

Adaptation 1:

Embracing Life Phases

Life changes, such as parenthood or career shifts, may impact your routine. Embrace these changes by adjusting your expectations and finding creative ways to stay active within your new lifestyle.

Adaptation 2:

Setting Realistic Goals

During busy periods, set realistic and achievable fitness goals. This might involve adjusting the frequency or duration of your workouts to align with your current priorities.

Adapting your fitness program for long-term success is not a sign of weakness but a testament to your commitment to sustained well-being. My journey in the 30-day Fat Burning Challenge underscored the dynamic nature of fitness. By incorporating individualized adjustments, embracing enjoyable activities, and periodically reassessing goals, you set the stage for a lifelong fitness journey.

Note... Remember, adaptation is not about compromising; it's about evolving and thriving. Keep sweating it out ...

CHAPTER 5: OVERCOMING COMMON CHALLENGES

5.1: CONSISTENCY , MINDSET and MOTIVATION

Embarking on a 30-day fat burning challenge is not just a physical journey; it's a mental and emotional one too. In this chapter, we'll delve into the importance of consistency, mindset, and motivation for total beginners without any equipment. Let's keep it straightforward and provide practical tips for building a strong foundation.

CONSISTENCY : The Bedrock of Success

1. Establishing Routine:

- Tip: Set a consistent workout schedule that fits into your daily life.

- Why: Routine builds habits, making it easier to stay committed to your fat-burning challenge.

2. Start Small, Build Gradually:

- Tip: Begin with manageable workouts and gradually increase intensity.

- Why: Small, consistent steps lay the groundwork for sustainable progress.

3. Accountability Matters:

- Tip: Find a workout buddy or join a community for mutual support.

- Why: Accountability fosters consistency and provides encouragement during challenging times.

4. Celebrate Small Wins:

- Tip: Acknowledge and celebrate each achievement, no matter how small.

- Why: Positive reinforcement reinforces the habit of consistency.

MINDSET : Shaping Your Approach to Fitness

1. Embrace the Journey:

- Mindset Shift: View your fat-burning challenge as a positive journey, not just a destination.

- Practical Tip: Focus on the joy of movement and the improvements you notice along the way.

2. Challenge Negative Thoughts:

- Practical Exercise: Identify and challenge negative thoughts about exercise.

- Why: Positive thoughts lead to a healthier mindset and increased motivation.

3. Be Kind to Yourself:

- Practical Tip: Replace self-criticism with self-compassion.

- Why: Treating yourself kindly fosters a positive relationship with your body and your fitness journey.

4. Adopt a Growth Mindset:

- Mindset Shift: Embrace challenges as opportunities for growth.

- Practical Tip: Instead of saying, "I can't do this," say, "I can't do this yet."

MOTIVATION: Fueling Your Fitness Drive

1. Find Your Why:

- Practical Exercise: Clearly define your reasons for undertaking the fat-burning challenge.

- Why: Understanding your motivations strengthens your commitment.

2. Visualize Your Goals:

- Practical Tip: Create a mental image of your fitness goals.

- Why: Visualization enhances motivation and helps you stay focused on your objectives.

3. Mix Up Your Routine:

- Tip: Introduce variety into your workouts to keep them interesting.

- Why: Novelty prevents boredom and rekindles motivation.

4. Create Incentives:

- Practical Tip: Establish rewards for reaching milestones.

- Why: Incentives provide tangible motivation and make the journey more enjoyable.

Practical Tips for Your 30-Day Fat Burning Challenge:

1. Daily Affirmations:

- Tip: Start each day with a positive affirmation related to your fitness journey.

- Why: Affirmations shape a positive mindset and set the tone for the day.

2. Set Realistic Expectations:

- Tip: Establish achievable short-term goals.

- Why: Realistic expectations reduce pressure and increase the likelihood of success.

3. Create a Motivational Playlist:

- Tip: Compile a playlist of energizing songs for your workouts.

- Why: Music enhances motivation and can make workouts more enjoyable.

4. Track Progress:

- Tip: Keep a record of your workouts and how you feel after each session.

- Why: Tracking progress provides a visual representation of your achievements.

5. Morning Visualization Routine:

- Practical Exercise: Spend a few minutes visualizing a successful workout.

- Why: Morning visualization sets a positive tone for the day ahead.

6. Flexible Mindset:

- Mindset Shift: Embrace adaptability in your fitness journey.

- Practical Tip: If a scheduled workout doesn't fit, find an alternative that does.

7. Reflect on Yourself:

- Tip: Regularly revisit and reflect on your initial motivations.

- Why: Connecting with your why reinforces your commitment during challenging moments.

8. Rest and Recovery Days:

- Tip: Schedule rest and recovery days into your routine.

- Why: Rest is a crucial part of the process, preventing burnout and supporting long-term consistency.

Navigating Consistency, Mindset, and Motivation:

Morning Routine:

- Start your day with a positive affirmation related to your fitness journey.

- Visualize yourself completing your workout successfully.

Pre-Workout:

- Remind yourself of the positive changes you're working towards.

- Listen to your favorite motivational music to energize your workout.

During Exercise:

- Challenge negative thoughts if they arise during challenging exercises.

- Celebrate small victories, whether it's completing an extra set or improving your form.

Post-Workout:

- Reflect on how the workout made you feel, both physically and mentally.

- Note any improvements or achievements, reinforcing a positive mindset.

Evening Routine:

- Set intentions for the next day's workout, focusing on your goals.

- Practice gratitude for the effort you've invested

in your fitness journey throughout the day.

CONCLUSION : Building a Strong Foundation for Success

Consistency, mindset, and motivation are the pillars that support your 30-day fat burning challenge. By establishing a routine, cultivating a positive mindset, and fueling your motivation, you're not just working on your body – you're shaping a holistic approach to health and well-being. Keep it simple, celebrate your progress, and remember that each day is an opportunity to grow stronger, both physically and mentally. As you navigate this journey, let the principles of consistency, a positive mindset, and unwavering motivation guide you towards lasting success in your 30-day fat burning challenge.

5.2: DEALING and OVERCOMING PlATEAUS

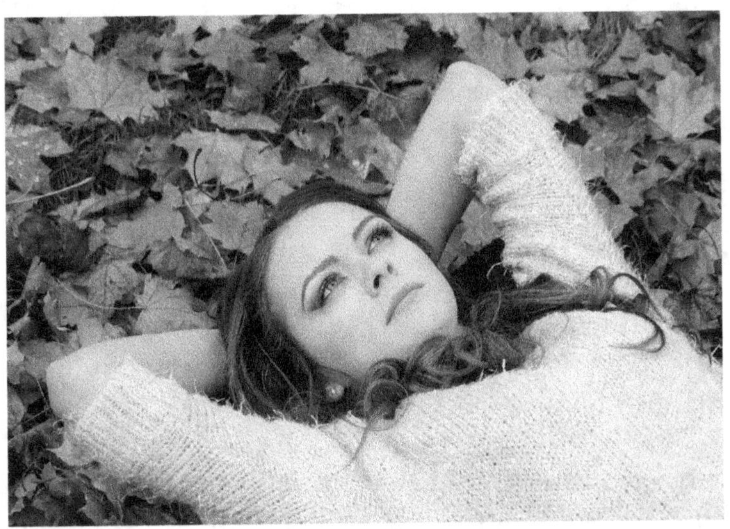

Encountering plateaus during your fitness journey is common, but overcoming them is where true progress lies. In this chapter, we'll explore practical strategies to navigate plateaus during a 30-day fat burning challenge for total beginners without any equipment. Let's keep it clear, simple, and equip you with the tools to push through.

Understanding Plateaus: Why They Happen

1. Your Body's Adaptation:

- Simple Explanation:Your body adapts to the exercises you've been doing, making them less challenging over time.

- Practical Insight: As your body becomes more efficient, it burns fewer calories during familiar workouts.

2. Routine Becomes Monotonous:

- Simple Explanation: Doing the same exercises every day can lead to boredom and reduced motivation.

- Practical Insight: Lack of variety may impact your engagement and effort during workouts.

3. Nutritional Habits Play a Role:

- Simple Explanation: Dietary habits can plateau, affecting your overall progress.

- Practical Insight: Evaluating and adjusting your nutrition is essential for continued success.

Practical Tips to Break Through Plateaus:

1. Mix Up Your Workouts:

- Tip: Introduce variety into your routine by trying new exercises.

- Why: Novelty challenges your muscles in different ways, preventing adaptation.

2. Adjust Intensity Levels:

- TIP: Gradually increase the intensity of your workouts.

- Why: Higher intensity challenges your body, leading to increased calorie burn.

3. Incorporate Strength Training:

- Tip: Add strength training exercises to build lean muscle mass.

- Why: Muscle burns more calories at rest, contributing to a higher metabolism.

4. High-Intensity Interval Training (HIIT):

- Tip: Include short bursts of high-intensity exercises in your routine.

- Why: HIIT can boost metabolism and break through plateaus effectively.

5. Evaluate Your Nutrition:

- Tip: Review your dietary habits and ensure you're consuming enough nutrients.

- Why: Proper nutrition fuels your workouts and supports overall progress.

6. Stay Hydrated:

- Tip: Ensure you're drinking enough water throughout the day.

- Why: Dehydration can impact performance and hinder progress.

7. Set New Goals:

- Tip: Establish fresh, achievable goals.

- Why: Goals provide motivation and direction, breaking the monotony of a plateau.

8. Monitor Your Rest and Recovery:

- Tip: Ensure you're getting adequate rest between workouts.

- Why: Proper recovery prevents burnout and supports sustained effort.

Navigating Plateaus Throughout Your 30-Day Challenge:

Week 1-2:

Establishing a Routine

- Initial enthusiasm is high, and progress is noticeable.

- Focus on learning proper form and building consistency.

Week 3-4:

Introducing Variety

- Incorporate new exercises to prevent early plateaus.

- Observe how your body responds to different movements.

Week 5-6:

Gradually Increasing Intensity

- Begin elevating the intensity of your workouts.

- Pay attention to your energy levels and adjust intensity accordingly.

Week 7-10:

Strength Training Emphasis

- Integrate strength training exercises into your routine.

- Track improvements in strength and endurance.

Week 11-14:

Incorporating HIIT Workouts

- Introduce HIIT sessions for a metabolic boost.

- Monitor how your body reacts to short bursts of high-intensity exercises.

Week 15-18: Nutrition Evaluation

- Assess your dietary habits and make adjustments as needed.

- Ensure you're fueling your body adequately for workouts.

Week 19-22:

Staying Hydrated

- Emphasize proper hydration throughout the day.

- Evaluate the impact of hydration on your energy levels.

Week 23-26:

Setting New Goals

- Establish fresh goals to keep motivation high.

- Celebrate achievements and acknowledge progress.

Week 27-30:

Monitoring Rest and Recovery

- Pay attention to signs of fatigue or burnout.

- Adjust your rest days as necessary to support recovery.

CONCLUSION : Breaking Through and Beyond

Plateaus are not roadblocks; they're opportunities for growth and adaptation. By incorporating variety, adjusting intensity, and paying attention to your nutrition and recovery, you empower yourself to break through plateaus during your 30-day fat burning challenge. Keep it simple, stay engaged, and remember that progress is a journey, not just a destination. As you navigate through challenges, your commitment, adaptability, and perseverance will carry you beyond plateaus, ensuring a fulfilling and successful fitness journey.

5.3: EMBRACING ADAPTABILITY

Adaptability is the secret sauce in any fitness journey, especially during a 30-day fat burning challenge. In this chapter, we'll explore the importance of being adaptable and provide practical tips for total beginners without any equipment. Let's keep it straightforward and equip you with the tools to navigate the twists and turns of your fitness adventure.

Understanding Adaptability: Why It Matters

1. Ever-Changing Circumstances:

   - Simple Insight: Life is unpredictable, and circumstances may vary from day to day.

   - Practical Consideration: Being adaptable allows you to adjust your fitness routine based on changing situations.

2. Physical Response to Workouts:

   - Simple Insight: Your body's response to exercises may differ, requiring adjustments.

- Practical Consideration: Adaptability ensures that your workouts remain effective and prevent plateaus.

3. Mental and Emotional Flexibility:

- Simple Insight: Your mindset and emotions play a crucial role in your fitness journey.

- Practical Consideration: Being adaptable helps you navigate challenges and setbacks without losing motivation.

Practical Tips for Embracing Adaptability:

1. Create a Flexible Workout Schedule:

- Tip: Have a general workout plan but be open to adjusting it based on your daily commitments.

- Why: Flexibility in your schedule ensures that you can always find time for exercise.

2. Alternate Between Workout Styles:

- Tip: Incorporate a mix of cardio, strength training, and flexibility exercises.

- Why: Switching between different workout styles prevents monotony and engages various muscle groups.

3. Listen to Your Body:

- Tip: Pay attention to how your body feels before, during, and after workouts.

- Why: Adapting based on your body's signals prevents overtraining and reduces the risk of injury.

4. Be Open to Modifications:

- Tip: Modify exercises to suit your current fitness level or address any physical limitations.

- Why: Adaptations ensure that you can perform exercises safely and consistently.

5. Adjust Intensity as Needed:

- Tip: Be willing to dial up or down the intensity of your workouts.

- Why: This allows you to match your energy levels and prevent burnout.

6. Explore Home-Friendly Workouts:

- Tip: Have a repertoire of home-friendly exercises for days when you can't make it to the gym.

- Why: Ensures that you have a backup plan for any situation.

7. Incorporate Short, Effective Workouts:

- Tip: On busy days, opt for shorter but high-intensity workouts.

- Why: Short workouts maintain consistency, keeping you on track even during hectic schedules.

8. Stay Positive During Setbacks:

- Tip: Maintain a positive mindset when facing obstacles or setbacks.

- Why: A positive outlook enhances adaptability and resilience in the face of challenges.

Navigating Adaptability Throughout Your 30-Day Challenge:

Week 1-2:

Establishing a Routine

- Create a basic workout schedule but remain open to adjustments.

- Explore different exercise styles to find what you enjoy.

Week 3-4:

Listening to Your Body

- Pay attention to how your body responds to workouts.

- Modify exercises or intensity levels based on your comfort and energy levels.

Week 5-6:

Exploring Home-Friendly Workouts

- Familiarize yourself with exercises that can be done at home.

- Use these as a backup plan on days when going to the gym is challenging.

Week 7-10:

Adapting to Time Constraints

- On busy days, opt for shorter but effective workouts.

- Prioritize consistency, even if it means adjusting your routine.

Week 11-14:

Adjusting Intensity Levels

- Evaluate your energy levels and adapt the intensity of your workouts accordingly.

- Ensure that your workouts remain challenging without causing excessive fatigue.

Week 15-18:

Staying Positive During Setbacks

- Maintain a positive mindset if you encounter setbacks.

- Adapt your approach, focus on solutions, and keep moving forward.

Week 19-22:

Alternating Workout Styles

- Combine cardiovascular, strength-training, and flexibility exercises.

- Adapt your routine based on what your body needs on a given day.

Week 23-26:

Openness to Modifications

- Modify exercises to accommodate any physical limitations or discomfort.

- Prioritize safety and consistent effort.

Week 27-30:

Celebrating Adaptability

- Reflect on how adaptability has been crucial in sustaining your fitness journey.

- Acknowledge your ability to navigate challenges and overcome obstacles.

CONCLUSION : Thriving in the Face of Change

Adaptability is your ally in the ever-changing landscape of a 30-day fat burning challenge. By creating a flexible workout schedule, listening to your body, and staying positive during setbacks, you're not just exercising your body – you're strengthening your ability to adapt and thrive. Keep it simple, stay open to adjustments, and let adaptability be the compass that guides you through your fitness journey, ensuring success beyond the 30-day mark.

5.4: MIND OVER MATTER

Unlocking the full potential of your 30-day fat burning challenge goes beyond physical effort—it's about mastering the mental game. In this chapter, we'll explore the powerful concept of "Mind Over Matter" and provide practical tips tailored for total beginners without any equipment. Let's keep it clear, straightforward, and equip you with the mental tools to conquer your fitness journey.

Understanding Mind Over Matter: The Power Within

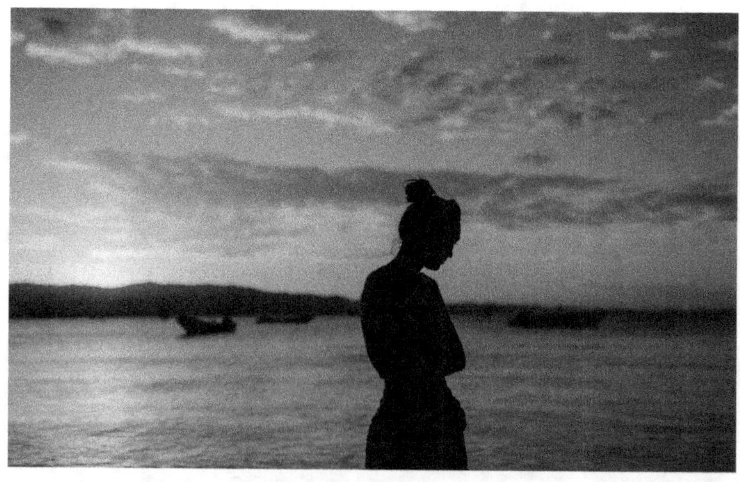

1. **Mindset Shapes Reality:**

- Simple Insight: Your thoughts influence your actions and, consequently, your results.

- Practical Consideration: Cultivating a positive mindset sets the stage for success in your fat-burning challenge.

2. **Overcoming Mental Barriers**:

- Simple Insight: Mental obstacles can hinder progress more than physical limitations.

- Practical Consideration: Developing mental resilience empowers you to push through challenges.

3. **Focus on the Present:**

- Simple Insight: Concentrating on the current moment enhances performance.

- Practical Consideration: Being present during workouts maximizes effort and engagement.

Practical Tips for Cultivating Mind Over Matter:

1. Set Clear Intentions:

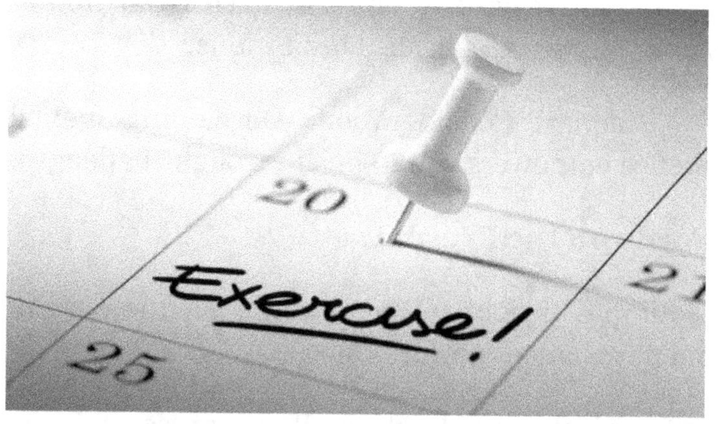

- Tip: Clearly define your goals and intentions for the 30-day challenge.

- Why: Clear objectives provide direction and motivation.

2. Positive Affirmations:

- Tip: Incorporate positive statements into your daily routine.

- Why: Affirmations shape a positive mindset and counteract self-doubt.

3. Visualize Success:

- Tip: Visualize yourself achieving your fitness goals.

- Why: Visualization enhances motivation and helps overcome mental barriers.

4. Develop a Mantra:

- Tip: Create a short, motivating phrase to repeat during challenging moments.

- Why: A mantra can refocus your mind and boost determination.

5. Practice Mindful Breathing:

- Tip: Integrate deep, mindful breaths into your workouts.

- Why:Controlled breathing reduces stress and enhances focus.

6. Break Down Big Goals:

- Tip: Divide larger goals into smaller, more manageable milestones.

-Why: Achieving smaller victories builds confidence and momentum.

7. Embrace Positivity:

- Tip: Surround yourself with positive influences.

- Why: Positivity from others and within yourself fosters a supportive environment.

8. Accept Imperfections:

- Tip: Understand that progress is not always linear, and setbacks happen.

- Why: Accepting imperfections prevents undue stress and helps maintain a positive mindset.

Navigating Mind Over Matter Throughout Your 30-Day Challenge:

Week 1-2: Setting Clear Intentions

- Define your goals for the 30-day challenge.

- Establish a positive mindset as you embark on your fitness journey.

Week 3-4: Introducing Positive Affirmations

- Incorporate daily affirmations into your routine.

- Notice how positive thoughts impact your motivation and approach to workouts.

Week 5-6: Visualizing Success

- Spend a few minutes each day visualizing successful workouts.

- Use visualization techniques to overcome mental barriers during exercises.

Week 7-10: Developing a Mantra

- Create a short, motivating phrase to use during challenging moments.

- Practice your mantra during high-intensity exercises or moments of fatigue.

Week 11-14: Mindful Breathing Techniques

- Integrate mindful breathing into your workouts.

- Pay attention to how controlled breathing enhances your focus and endurance.

Week 15-18: Breaking Down Big Goals

- Divide larger fitness goals into smaller, achievable milestones.

- Celebrate each small victory, reinforcing a positive mindset.

Week 19-22: Embracing Positivity

- Surround yourself with positive influences, whether from friends, family, or online communities.

- Share your achievements and receive encouragement from others.

Week 23-26: Accepting Imperfections

- Understand that setbacks may occur, and progress is not always linear.

- Approach challenges with a solutions-oriented mindset.

- Share your fitness journey with others, spreading positivity and motivation.

- Actively engage in supportive communities to foster a sense of camaraderie.

Week 27-30: Reflecting on Mind Over Matter

- Reflect on how cultivating a positive mindset impacted your fitness journey.

- Carry the mental tools you've developed into the post-30-day phase.

- Reflect on setbacks not as failures but as opportunities for learning.

- Adjust your approach based on the lessons learned during challenges.

Integrating Mind Over Matter into Your Daily Routine:

Morning Routine:

- Start your day with a positive affirmation related to your fitness journey.

- Visualize the successful completion of your workout for the day.

Pre-Workout:

- Recite your motivating mantra to boost your mental readiness.

- Practice mindful breathing to center yourself before diving into exercise.

During Exercise:

- Use visualization to conquer mental barriers during challenging moments.

- Repeat positive affirmations to maintain motivation and focus.

Post-Workout:

- Reflect on the mental and emotional benefits of your workout.

- Celebrate your commitment and effort, reinforcing a positive mindset.

Evening Routine:

- Acknowledge the achievements of the day, no matter how small.

- Incorporate relaxation techniques to promote a positive mindset before sleep.

Evolving Beyond the 30-Day Mark:

1. Continuous Goal Setting:

- Next Step: Extend your fitness goals beyond the initial 30 days.

- Why: Setting new objectives ensures a continued sense of purpose and progression.

2. Mindfulness as a Lifestyle:

- Next Step: Integrate mindful practices into your daily life.

- Why: Cultivating mindfulness contributes to overall well-being beyond your fitness journey.

3. Periodic Reflections:

- Next Step: Schedule regular reflections on your mental and physical well-being.

- Why: Reflection fosters self-awareness and guides ongoing personal growth.

4. Adaptability in Long-Term Fitness:

- Next Step: Embrace adaptability as a constant companion in your fitness journey.

- Why: Being adaptable ensures sustainability and prevents stagnation.

5. Sharing Your Journey:

- Next Step: Continue sharing your experiences with others.

- Why: Your journey can inspire and support others on their paths to a healthier lifestyle.

CONCLUSION : The Mind-Body Connection

In your 30-day fat burning challenge, your mental resilience is as crucial as your physical effort. By setting clear intentions, embracing positivity, and practicing mindfulness, you're not just exercising your body but nurturing the powerful connection between mind and matter. Keep it simple, focus on the present, and let the strength of your mindset propel you toward lasting success in your fitness journey beyond the 30-day mark.

Moving forward, let the lessons learned in these 30 days guide you toward enduring success, making mindfulness an integral part of your fitness and well-being journey.

5.5: PLANNING YOUR NEXT FITNESS JOURNEY

As you approach the end of your 30-day fat burning challenge, it's time to set the stage for what comes next. This chapter will guide you in planning your subsequent fitness journey, offering practical tips for total beginners without any equipment. Let's keep it clear, straightforward, and equip you with the tools to continue your fitness success beyond the initial challenge.

Reflecting on Your 30-Day Journey:

1. Celebrate Achievements:

- Reflection Point: Acknowledge and celebrate the milestones you've reached.

- Why: Celebrating achievements boosts motivation and creates a positive outlook.

2. Learn from Challenges:

- Reflection Point: Reflect on the challenges you encountered and how you overcame them.

- Why: Learning from challenges provides valuable insights for future planning.

3. Assess What Worked:

- Reflection Point: Identify the exercises, routines, and habits that were most effective.

- Why: Knowing what worked well helps you build on successful strategies.

Setting New Fitness Goals

1. Define Clear Objectives:

- Tip: Establish specific and measurable fitness goals for the next phase.

- Why: Clear objectives provide direction and motivation.

2. Consider Diverse Fitness Aspects:

- Tip: Include goals related to strength, endurance, flexibility, and overall well-being.

- Why: Diversifying your goals ensures a balanced approach to fitness.

3. Gradual Progression:

- Tip: Set goals that challenge you but are attainable with consistent effort.

- Why: Gradual progression prevents burnout and encourages sustainable growth.

Choosing Your Workout Routine:

1. Explore New Exercises:

   - Tip: Introduce fresh exercises to keep your routine interesting.

   - Why: Variety prevents boredom and engages different muscle groups.

2. Incorporate Strength Training:

   - Tip: Continue integrating strength training for overall fitness.

   - Why: Building muscle enhances metabolism and contributes to fat burning.

3. Mix Cardio and High-Intensity Workouts:

   - Tip: Combine cardio sessions with high-intensity interval training (HIIT).

   - Why: This combination maximizes calorie burn and improves cardiovascular health.

Planning Your Weekly Schedule:

1. Set a Realistic Routine:

   - Tip: Create a weekly workout schedule that aligns with your daily commitments.

   - Why: Realistic routines are easier to maintain, fostering consistency.

2. Include Rest Days:

   - Tip: Schedule designated rest days to allow your body proper recovery.

   - Why: Adequate rest prevents burnout and reduces the risk of overtraining.

3. Flexibility in Your Plan:

   - Tip: Allow for flexibility in your schedule to adapt to unexpected changes.

   -Why: Adaptability ensures you can stick to your plan even during busy times.

Nutritional Considerations:

1. Evaluate Your Dietary Habits:

- Tip: Reflect on your eating habits during the previous challenge.

- Why: Understanding your nutrition helps align it with your fitness goals.

2. Hydration Focus:

- Tip: Prioritize staying hydrated throughout the day.

- Why: Hydration is essential for overall health and supports your fitness efforts.

3. Mindful Eating Practices:

- Tip: Practice mindful eating by savoring each bite and paying attention to hunger cues.

- Why: Mindful eating fosters a healthier relationship with food.

Incorporating Mindfulness:

1. Continue Mental Resilience Practices:

- Tip: Carry forward mental tools like positive affirmations and visualization.

- Why: Mindfulness contributes to both mental and physical well-being.

2. Settle into Mindful Workouts:

- Tip: Maintain mindfulness during workouts by focusing on each movement.

- Why: Being present enhances the effectiveness of your exercises.

3. Mindfulness Beyond Workouts:

- Tip: Extend mindfulness practices into your daily life, promoting overall balance.

- Why: Mindfulness supports stress management and a positive mindset.

Creating a Supportive Environment:

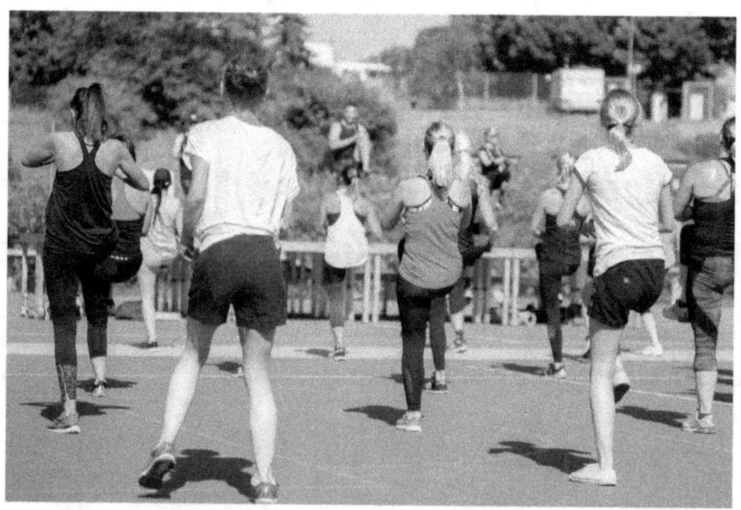

1. Engage with Fitness Communities:

  - Tip: Join online or local fitness communities to stay motivated.

  - Why: Sharing experiences and receiving encouragement fosters a supportive environment.

2. Involve Friends or Family:

  - Tip: Encourage friends or family members to join your fitness journey.

  - Why: Having workout buddies adds a social element and increases accountability.

Preparing for Long-Term Success:

1. Commit to Consistency:

  - Next Step: Prioritize consistency in your fitness routine.

  - Why: Consistency is the key to long-term success and lasting health benefits.

2. Embrace Continuous Learning:

  - Next Step: Stay informed about fitness trends, nutrition, and wellness.

- Why: Continuous learning ensures you can adapt your approach based on new information.

3. Celebrate Milestones Along the Way:

- Next Step: Set smaller milestones and celebrate them regularly.

- Why: Regular celebrations reinforce your commitment and provide positive reinforcement.

CONCLUSION: Your Fitness Journey Continues

As you embark on planning your next fitness journey, remember that it's a continuation rather than a conclusion. Reflect on your achievements, set clear goals, diversify your workouts, and foster a supportive environment. With a realistic plan, a mindful approach, and a commitment to consistency, your fitness journey becomes a lifelong adventure filled with health, vitality, and the joy of continuous growth. Congratulations on completing your 30-day fat burning challenge, and here's to the exciting chapters that lie ahead in your fitness story!

CHAPTER 6: FREQUENTLY ASKED QUESTIONS (FAQs)

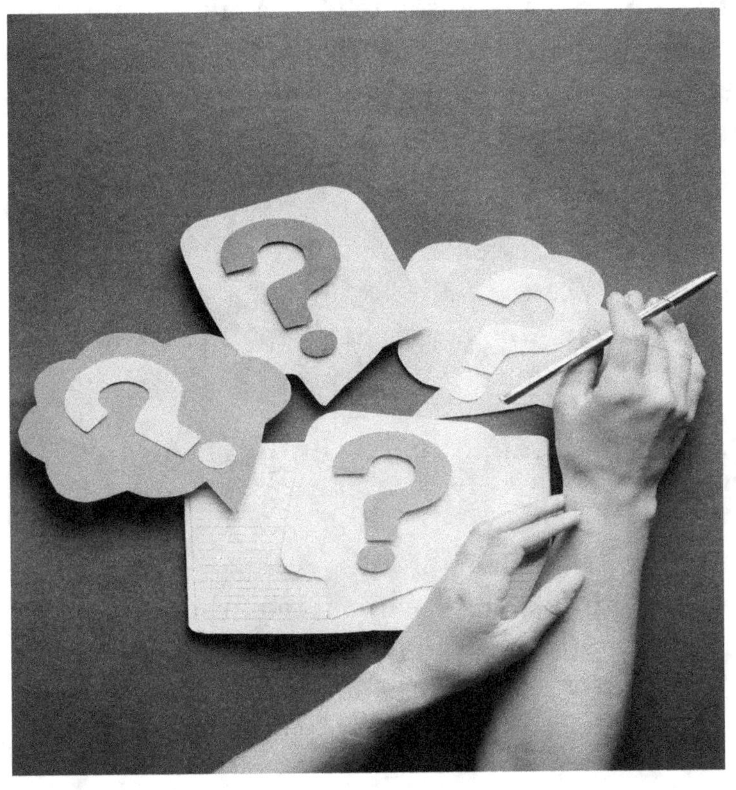

Embarking on a 30-day fat burning challenge as a total beginner can spark numerous questions. Let's address some of the most common inquiries to ensure you have a clear and confident start to your fitness journey.

Q1: Can I Really See Results in 30 Days as a Beginner?

Answer: Yes, absolutely! While significant transformations may vary individually, many beginners witness noticeable improvements in strength, endurance, and overall fitness within 30 days. Consistency and commitment are key.

Tip: Set realistic goals, celebrate small victories, and trust the process. Progress may not always be visible on the scale; focus on how you feel and your increased stamina.

Q2: Do I Need Special Equipment for the Challenge?

Answer: Not at all! This 30-day challenge is designed for beginners without requiring any special equipment. Bodyweight exercises can be highly effective, and you can perform them in the comfort of your home.

Tip: Ensure you have a comfortable workout space with enough room to move. A yoga mat can add comfort but is not essential.

Q3: Is It Normal to Feel Soreness?

Answer: Yes, it's completely normal, especially for beginners. This muscle soreness, known as delayed onset muscle soreness (DOMS), indicates that your muscles are adapting to new movements.

Tip: Stay hydrated, stretch before and after workouts, and consider incorporating rest days to allow your muscles to recover.

Q4: How Many Rest Days Should I Take?

Answer: Rest days are crucial for recovery. Depending on your fitness level and personal preferences, aim for at least one or two rest days per week. Pay attention to your body and make necessary adjustments.

Tip: Use rest days for light activities like walking or gentle stretching to promote recovery without intense workouts.

Q5: Can I Modify Exercises if They're Too Challenging?

Answer: Absolutely! Modification is a great approach for beginners. If an exercise feels too challenging, simplify it or reduce the intensity. The key is to maintain proper form and gradually progress.

Tip: Focus on building a strong foundation with proper form before advancing to more challenging variations.

Q6: How Should I Handle Days When I Lack Motivation?

Answer: Motivational slumps are normal. On such days, start with a shorter workout or choose activities you enjoy. Remember that consistency is more important than intensity.

Tip: Find a workout buddy, vary your routine, or set small, achievable goals to reignite motivation.

Q7: What Role Does Nutrition Play in the Challenge?

Answer: Nutrition is crucial for overall well-being and can complement your fitness efforts. Consume a balanced diet with a mix of protein, carbohydrates, and healthy fats. Stay hydrated for optimal performance.

Tip:Pay attention to portion sizes, include a variety of whole foods, and consider consulting a nutritionist for personalized guidance.

Q8: Can I Continue the Challenge Beyond 30 Days?

Answer: Absolutely! The 30-day challenge is a great starting point, but your fitness journey doesn't end there. Consider setting new goals, exploring different workout styles, and making exercise a consistent part of your lifestyle.

Tip: Reflect on your achievements, adjust your goals, and continue building on the momentum you've gained.

Q9: What if I Miss a Day or Two of Workouts?

Answer: It happens! Don't be too hard on yourself. Simply pick up where you left off even if you miss a day or two. Consistency over the long term matters more than perfection.

Tip: Use missed days as a chance to reassess your schedule and make adjustments for better consistency.

Q10: How Do I Stay Consistent Beyond the Challenge?

Answer: Consistency is a gradual process. Set a realistic schedule, find activities you enjoy, and involve friends or family for added accountability. Celebrate your successes along the way.

Tip: Create a fitness routine that aligns with your lifestyle, making it easier to maintain in the long run.

CONCLUSION: Your Questions, Your Journey

As you embark on this 30-day fat burning challenge, your questions are not obstacles but stepping stones to a successful fitness journey. Embrace the learning process, celebrate every achievement, and remember that everyone's path is unique. Keep your focus on progress, stay consistent, and enjoy the transformative journey you've set upon. Here's to your health, strength, and the fulfillment of your fitness goals!

CONCLUSION

For a while, take a moment to reflect on the incredible journey we have embarked on together, this journey has been about more than sets, reps, fitness or diet and reaching fitness milestones. It's been a quest to understand that true wellness isn't a destination but a daily commitment to our well-being.

We've explored the power of mindset, the importance of balanced nutrition, the significance of diverse workouts, and the often-overlooked heroes of rest and recovery. Each chapter has been a stepping stone, guiding you towards a holistic approach to a healthier you.

As you close this book, remember that it's not about perfection but progress. Celebrate the small victories, embrace the setbacks as lessons, and relish the journey. Fitness is a lifelong adventure, and you're the protagonist.

The call to action is clear: take what you've learned here and make it a part of your lifestyle.

-Set realistic goals.

-be kind to yourself.

-cultivate a mindset of consistency.

-Apply the principles of balanced nutrition, varied workouts.

-Always rest in your daily routine.

Note.... It's not about a 30-day sprint; it's about the lifelong marathon of well-being.

Your body is capable of incredible things, and each day is a new opportunity to nurture it. So, rise to the challenge, step into your strength, and let this be a starting point for a healthier, happier, and more fulfilled version of yourself.

Thank you for being a part of this journey. Here's to the next chapter – your journey to a vibrant and energized life. Keep moving, stay motivated, and let your well-being be your greatest achievement. **The adventure continues – make it extraordinary!**

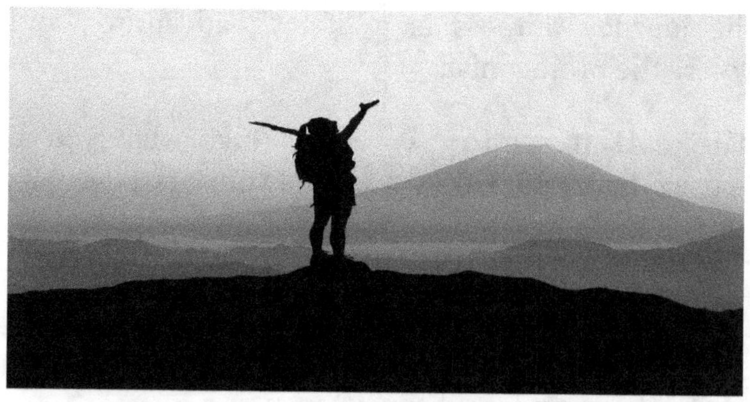

www.ingramcontent.com/pod-product-compliance
Lightning Source LLC
Chambersburg PA
CBHW050809260726

48660CB00004B/1340